WAYNE PERRY

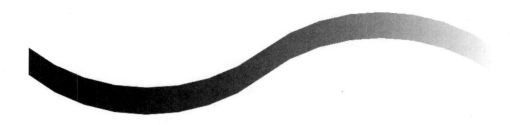

SOUND MEDICINE

*The Complete Guide to Healing
With the Human Voice*

NEW PAGE BOOKS
A division of The Career Press, Inc.
Franklin Lakes, NJ

Copyright © 2007 by Wayne Perry
All rights reserved under the Pan-American and International Copyright Conventions.
This book may not be reproduced, in whole or in part, in any form or by any means
electronic or mechanical, including photocopying, recording, or by any information
storage and retrieval system now known or hereafter invented, without written
permission from the publisher, The Career Press.

SOUND MEDICINE
EDITED BY JODI BRANDON
TYPESET BY EILEEN DOW MUNSON
Cover design by Scott Fray
Printed in the U.S.A. by Book-mart Press
To order this title, please call toll-free 1-800-CAREER-1 (NJ and Canada: 201-848-
0310) to order using VISA or MasterCard, or for further information on books from
Career Press.

Disclaimer From the Publisher and Author

Any information given in this book is not intended to be taken as a replacement
for medical advice. Any person with a condition requiring medical attention should
consult a qualified practitioner, physician, or other healthcare professional.

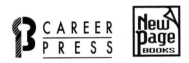

The Career Press, Inc., 3 Tice Road, PO Box 687,
Franklin Lakes, NJ 07417
www.careerpress.com
www.newpagebooks.com

Library of Congress Cataloging-in-Publication Data
Perry, Wayne, 1946–
    Sound medicine: the complete guide to healing with the human voice / by Wayne
Perry.
        p. cm.
    Includes bibliographical references and index.
    ISBN-13: 978-1-56414-970-1
    ISBN-10: 1-56414-970-6
    1. Sound—Therapeutic use. 2. Singing—Therapeutic use. 3. Vibration
(Therapeutics) 4. Music therapy. I. Title.

RZ999.P47 2007
615.8'5154--dc22

                                                                    2007042598

If the eyes are the windows to the soul,
the voice is surely the door to the heart.

For "old soul" Nicole

Acknowledgments ~

First and foremost, my heartfelt thanks to all the kindred spirits, friends, colleagues, clients, teachers, and students who have touched, motivated, and inspired me through your courage, faith, and willingness to love and heal yourselves. Although too numerous to mention all of you by name, you know who you are. And you are truly the "keepers of the tone" and the "voices of the future."

I do feel compelled to acknowledge the love and friendship I've received from some of my spiritual brothers and sisters. They include my beloved Sammie and Moreah Love, Bruce and Shari Silvey, Steve and Sheryl Robinson, Doug Gordon, Michael Dunn, Jackie Calamos, Lee Silver, Glenn Woodside, Phil Wilson, Jeff Fetzer, and my Pittsburgh buddies: Michael Jon and Glenn Freund. You've all touched my life in unique and special ways.

I greatly love and appreciate my precious and loving daughter Brittany, for your presence in my life. Your sweet soul has been a source of joy and support since the day you were born. My son-in-law, Tom, for your solid support and pure heart. And my brothers Bruce and Frank for your friendship, honesty, and humor.

Very special thanks to my beautiful "fairy goddess" Nicole, my so sweet and patient wife, friend, "harmonic," and life partner, who ceaselessly showers me with unconditional love and unflagging devotion. Your wisdom, purity, and integrity fill my life with purpose and joy.

My appreciation and respect to my editors, Cynthia Crossman and Gina Hillier, for your professional expertise and guidance. Michele DeFilippo and your design team for beautiful graphics artistry in the book's cover and interior. And thanks to Craig Lund for your computer graphic services and longtime support.

For inspiring me on my journey with the voice, I am grateful to Sharry Edwards's pioneering sound work with bio-acoustics and the voice; Jonathan Goldman for his knowledge of healing sounds and harmonics; Florence Riggs for her big heart and vocal spirit; and Bobby McFerrin, Al Jarreau, and Tim Buckley, whose extraordinary vocal creativity touched me at the right times and helped teach me to trust my voice. And particularly to my mom for all the songs she sang to me from her heart when I was a boy. Love resonations!

Special mention deserves to be made for Arnold Patent, for his insightful teachings on love and universal principles. Sincere thanks for the inspired leadership of John Gray, Michael Beckwith, and Jim Quinn, who greatly influenced me as mentors. And my dad, who taught me responsibility and devotion.

Finally, words cannot express the profound gratitude I hold in my heart for my beloved spiritual teacher and "mystic mentor," Huzur Charan Singh, who was the embodiment of love, service, and humility. And to his devoted successor Gurinder Singh, and all the "living" masters of the Sound Current and Inner Overtone who are One in Spirit. Radha Soami!

$(((((\bullet)))))$

Contents

≈

Exercises

$(((((\bullet)))))$

Preface

As I've reflected from time to time on my life's interests, studies, and work, I've always found them inextricably connected to my voice. From the age of 5 when I began singing at family wedding receptions (getting paid one dollar from my uncle!), through years of performing, recording, and radio and television hosting, the effective use of the voice has always been vital to my success. And now in my current service of teaching, lecturing, and seminar facilitating on sound therapy, toning, and vocal vibrational healing, the voice is still "center stage."

Upon discovering the role and value that sound, frequency, and vibration play in vocal expression, my interest in the voice began to expand from the purely auditory to the vibrationally pure. It gradually became evident to me that if I wanted to fully realize and express all the dimensions available in the voice, I needed to first gain access to the mysterious vibrational power of the inner voice. Only then would I be able to truly voice my soul.

Voicing the Soul

This may be an apt description of other soulful expressions as well. In the spiritual traditions of various cultures throughout time, the sacred power of devotional songs, chants, and mantras lies in the purity of that inner connection. It is this same Divine relationship with our real Soul-Self that can truly move and inspire us, and can touch others through us. This "soul-full" relationship is at the foundation of *Sound Medicine*.

However, words and books can take us only so far. They can be great tools for gathering information, learning, inspiration, and motivation. But it is we who must accept responsibility and take action. We must set the course, helm the ship, set sail, and embark on our journey. It is also we who, ultimately, sink or swim, succeed or fail, reach the destination and receive the rewards for our efforts.

The wise Greek philosopher Socrates once said, "Know thyself." An important admonition, no doubt, but we must know the true self. The real self is not merely an impermanent physical body, mind, and ephemeral self, but the permanent, pure-essence, Divine Soul-Self. To indeed know this Real Self, we must have a committed intention to honestly open up and love ourselves. We must have a working knowledge of universal truths and spiritual principles. This process may require guidance and practice, but it is available to everyone and need not be difficult.

Only through the conscious journey of "inner-acting" regularly with our Soul-Self can we begin to perceive and recognize the Soul-Self in all other "selves." When we act and communicate with our Real Self—by voicing the soul—we become an open channel for the Divine Spirit, Sacred Sound Current, or Infinite Overtone to create and express through us.

Voicing the soul is not just a method or technique. Methodology and practice are important, but at some point there must be surrender to Spirit so that the Soul-Self may be accessed and the inner voice released. Voicing the soul is an experience. And it's an experience that is available to everyone. Voicing the soul is also a direct expression of that experience.

Though there are certainly principles, practices, and techniques—on which this book intends to elaborate—that will assist you in achieving this experience, it is already within you. Voicing your soul is your birthright. It may even be your life's purpose.

Sound Questions and Answers

For the last 20 years or so, I have felt inspired by and compelled to write about this subject. But every time I put pen to paper I felt daunted and humbled by the enormity and profound importance of the topic. These feelings led to questions, such as: *Who am I to write about vibrational healing principles, spirituality, or even the human voice? What gives me the authority to instruct others on how to transform their lives? Am I truly "walking my talk," or somehow deluding myself?* These types of questions vibrated through my mind.

However, one of the most vital principles I learned on my healing journey is that everything—and I mean everything—we need exists within us. I discovered that I had to release my doubts and self-judgments, quiet my mind, and listen to the inner voice that kept telling me I would receive the guidance I needed. I was told to write from my heart and soul, get my mind and ego out of the way, and just be an open channel for whatever truths and information needed to come through. I have since tried my best to live my life this way as well.

Nevertheless, the five-year process of writing this book was a daunting task. It was also a great exercise in staying focused, disciplining myself, defining my path, and keeping my soul inspired. In retrospect, the writing was a profoundly healing experience. I hope it may in some way contribute to your unfolding transformation as well.

Throughout my experience of researching and writing *Sound Medicine*, I surrendered to the spirit of the principles contained within these pages and have diligently practiced the related exercises. I know that these spiritual and vibrational principles work. Their extraordinary power is not based on a belief; it is a knowing. I know that we all have a spiritual and vibrational power within us, but that for most this may be virtually unexplored because of our beliefs and conditioning. And I know that if you practice the methodology outlined in this book, you can begin to immediately experience the benefits and resonant results in your daily life. You will discover the remarkable healing capacity of your own voice. You will dramatically enhance health and wellness with the transformative power of sound. You can even, ultimately, transcend the limitations of mind and matter and experience the liberation of the soul with the discovery of the Inner Overtone.

In the years since discovering vibrational healing and the unique power of vocal overtoning, I've had several profound and effective self-healing experiences. By experimenting with this phenomenon, I've successfully healed several of my chronic disorders—including allergies, knee pain, and kidney stones (which I will talk about in later chapters).

Remember the Future

In the spring of 1992, a most unexpected, yet inspiring and precursory event drew me nearer to my purpose of voicing my soul. At the time, I was producing and hosting "Heart Touch," a radio program in Los Angeles dedicated to exploring leading-edge concerns and new-thought perspectives. I had just finished conducting an interview with "futurist" Gordon-Michael Scallion, renowned for his metaphysical insights and ability to forecast changes in the Earth's environment with a high degree of accuracy. Mr. Scallion bases his various predictions on what he calls "hits," or premonitory visions of future events, which he claims to literally see on a psychic screen in front of him. He states that his regular outer vision is actually temporarily blocked while these hits appear to him on his "inner viewing" screen.

Following his appearance on my radio show, I was invited to accompany Gordon, his wife, and a few of their friends for dinner at a nearby restaurant. After our meal we all sat for a while and talked. Suddenly, while speaking to the person across from him, Gordon stopped in mid-sentence and exclaimed, "I'm getting a hit on something!" We anxiously looked in his direction. He then stated what sounded to be, "It's about Wayne!" I almost fell out of my chair. Is he talking about me, I wondered? Did he really say Wayne? Did I hear him correctly? Was this a joke?

I recalled Gordon explaining earlier on my show that he has no control over when and where these hits take place. He even mentioned that, if it occurs while driving, he has to immediately pull over and stop the vehicle. And he never knows how long they will last. We all sat patiently transfixed, as Gordon sat quietly in a trance-like state.

In a few minutes he seemed to "return," and I anxiously asked him what he had seen. Gordon paused, his brow furrowed reflectively, and asked me if I teach or speak to large groups of people. I thought for a moment and replied that, hopefully, a large number of people were tuning into my radio show. Shaking his head, he said no. In his vision he had clearly seen me onstage before hundreds, or perhaps even thousands, of people. Because I sang and performed with my band at the time, I inquired if it could have been a musical performance he had seen. Gordon again replied no; he didn't think so. I appeared to be standing alone and merely speaking, but he said a brilliant white light was emanating from my throat!

I felt a chill immediately run through my body upon hearing his words. Everyone at the table sat in rapt attention. Gordon then said he saw the people in the audience moved, uplifted, and healed in some way by my voice and this "light" in it! Another chill rippled through me.

I wondered if there was any reality in what he said. In preparing for my various radio shows, I had received many personal readings and assorted predictions, and would routinely take them with a grain of salt. However, Gordon's forecast felt quite different. I had never experienced these chills before, and something inside me—though slightly confused and a bit skeptical—intuitively felt that there was more to this.

Little did I know at the time that within mere weeks of that fateful experience, to my surprise and delight, I would begin discovering the secrets to the healing power that lies within the human voice.

P ART I

A Sound Foundation

All matter consists of vibrating waveforms of energy. And though it may not be audible to the human ear, sound is emitted from these waveforms.

(((((1)))))

Inner-Duction

inner—of or relating to the mind or spirit

duct—a pipe or channel that conveys a substance

—*Webster's Seventh New Collegiate Dictionary*

inner-duction—the act or process of channeling or conveying something of substance for the mind or spirit

You have within your body the power and support of the Sound Current or "Inner Overtone." Throughout the ages, spiritual sages and masters have referred to this Sacred Sound as the Word, Logos, Om, Kalma, Shabd, Nam, Nada, Celestial Melody, Inner Voice, and other names. This Infinite Tone resonates within each one of us—sustaining life and offering true soul freedom and transcendence.

You also have within your voice a sonic means to vibrationally activate, heal, and harmonize body, mind, and spirit. When generated with intention from the heart and soul, the voice can be a miraculous and transformative tool of sound, light, and love. So the voice is not only the door to the heart, but can also express the song of the soul.

Toning

The nonverbal process of using the voice to assist in the harmonizing and healing of the body is commonly referred to as *toning*. The practice of toning uses various sounds created by the voice—without coherent meaning or reliance on the structural patterns of speaking or singing—to generate vibrational energy. When we sigh, grunt, groan, or hum to release stress, we tone routinely without necessarily realizing or calling it so. Toning can be used as an extraordinary tool for healing and transformation.

In her 1973 book, *Toning: The Creative Power of the Voice*, which may have been the first book published on the subject, Laurel Elizabeth Keyes writes, "Toning is an ancient method of healing, which I hope will be recognized and used with new understanding now that we have more scientific explanations for it." I hold the same hope now. And in my travels conducting toning seminars, I've noticed the interest and awareness of toning consistently growing worldwide.

Belief in the healing capacity of the voice has existed for ages within numerous cultures and throughout many parts of the world. Mystics and shamans use the sound of the voice to commune with higher consciousness. Primitive healers and medicine men used vocal sounds to stimulate spiritual and emotional cleansing in restoring health to the physical body.

The vowel sounds are the most dynamic aspect of vocal sound, for contained within them is the regenerative power of overtones. Together with the prana energy of breath, the vowel tones can open and harmonize various inner regions of the mind-body. In *Sound Medicine*, Laeh Maggie Garfield writes, "Toning is a system of healing that utilizes vowel sounds to alter vibrations in every molecule and cell in the body." Also addressing the healing capabilities of the human voice, Mitchell L. Gaynor, M.D., states in *Sounds of Healing*, "In my own sound/healing work, I have been profoundly influenced by toning practices...."

Overtoning

The most significant and profound facet of toning is *overtoning*, because it involves the creation of simultaneous, multiple tones referred to as *vocal overtones* and *harmonics* (the two terms may be used interchangeably). These innate "sounds within sounds" give the voice its timbre and tonal colors, but—more importantly—they effectively concentrate and activate the vibrational energy in the sound.

Overtoning is a remarkable vocal technique that requires no singing or musical experience, only a dedication to properly learn the practice involved. Overtoning can also be a useful method for extending and expanding the unique vibrational capabilities of the human voice. For example, when we focus our attention on the expression of overtones, they may be vocally projected into particular areas of the body—or the body of another—for healing. This intention and process is the essence of overtoning. (The principles and techniques involved in this potent, vibrational healing methodology are addressed in more detail later in this book.)

The powerful practice of vocal overtoning may also be used with an intention for enhancing spiritual growth and awareness. Laurel Elizabeth Keyes writes, "The voice belongs to the body and is its instrument. We, being more than the body, should use it as a tool for higher consciousness." And in *Healing Sounds*, my friend and colleague Jonathan Goldman writes, "From a physiological viewpoint, vocal harmonics create changes in the heartbeat, respiration and brainwaves of the reciter, altering consciousness and allowing the shaman to be in a state where they are receptive to spirit journeys."

The Power of Sacred Sound

For ages, ancient masters have stressed the importance of chanting or vocalizing sounds, mantras, and names of God for spiritual realization. For example, in his yoga sutras, Patanjali recommended repeating the "AUM" or "OM" sound to bypass the mind, release obstacles, access creative energy, and awaken to a higher consciousness.

Tibetan Buddhist monks combine mantric formulas with a type of overtoning called **throat-singing**, which allows the monks to be one with sacred sound and embody its energies.

In 1975, a friend gifted me with a wonderful and spiritually insightful book: *The Sufi Message of Hazrat Inayat Khan*. Actually a series of four books compiled from lectures given by the Sufi sound master between 1921 and 1937, this wealth of information on sacred sound and mysticism has been a great influence and inspiration in my life. In it, Inayat Khan says, "Very few in this world know to what extent phenomena can be produced by the power of voice. If there is any real trace of miracle, of phenomenon, of wonder, it is in the voice."

Sound Healing

Through the spring and summer of 1992, and shortly after my precognitive experience with Gordon-Michael Scallion, I enthusiastically studied available sound therapy research. I interviewed those working in this exciting field, and I talked with those who had received healing benefits from various types of sound healing. (A number of these experiences—including my own—are elaborated on in Part III and Part IV of this book.)

Before discovering the natural and profound healing capabilities of the human voice, I invested time and money in developing my skills with sound machines in the hope of achieving vibrationally therapeutic benefits. For five or six months, I freely offered my services to anyone desirous of exploring some "sound alternatives" to wellness. Many received improvement with their health issues, and I learned much through this experience.

Being inspired by the results and benefits that I, and others, received from sound healing, I entered professionally into the field of sound therapy and vibrational healing. Shortly thereafter, deciding that my healing experiences might help others—and feeling more comfortable using my voice than my pen—I recorded "The Ultimate Healing Instrument: THE HUMAN VOICE," an instructional recording containing the most effective practices I had developed in my own healing process.

I subsequently received a lot of favorable feedback from people all across the country who used these principles and techniques in healing themselves and improving the quality of their lives. This acknowledgment and validation inspired me to make several more recordings and finally compile this information, along with new material, into this book.

As mentioned earlier, the central theme of *Sound Medicine* is the use of vocal overtoning to assist in establishing homeostasis in the body, improving overall health and wellness, and preparing the mind-body for spiritual consciousness through sacred sound.

Throughout this book we will explore important and efficacious vibrational healing practices. I will also endeavor to explain, clarify, and demystify this comprehensive topic. Irrespective of your level of experience, with careful study and applied practice you will learn the skills necessary to achieve the transformative benefits of vocal overtoning. But be warned: You may sometimes feel vibrations of silliness and frequencies of fun in the process!

Other related subject matter to be discussed include:

≈ The mechanics, control, development, and creative use of the human voice.

≈ Accessing and developing the power of intuition and the Inner Voice.

≈ Ways in which you may discover, heal, and tune your own personal vibration and unique signature frequency.

≈ How personal relationships are attracted, impacted, and affected by each individual's vibrational signature, and how these frequencies determine relationship chemistry.

≈   The use of subtle-energy alternatives such as light and color frequencies, brainwave and sonic entrainment, resonance, polarities, astrology, and dowsing.

≈   The nature of the mind, ego, left- and right-brain influences, chakras, energy vortices, dimensions, time and space, reality, consciousness, and human awareness.

≈   Sonic meditation as a healing and harmonizing method for supporting the body, concentrating the mind, and uplifting the spirit.

≈   The spiritual power of the Inner Overtone or Sacred Sound Current.

Are You Out of Your Mind?

When executed properly, this methodology will assist you in going out of your mind. Fear not! This is one of your goals. We must ultimately leave the limitations of the finite mind for the freedom of the infinite spirit. Through the finer development of your unique signature frequency and soul's intuition, you can view the whole of your reality. You will then begin to access the clarity born of spiritual awareness and inner experience.

> *Through the finer development of your unique signature frequency and soul's intuition, you can view the whole of your reality.*

These are not "airy-fairy" pipe dreams, "pie-in-the-sky" speculations, or "New Age mumbo jumbo." They involve practical and focused methods. Although not easily quantifiable, true vibrational principles and practices lead one to universal truths and achievable transformation.

> *True vibrational principles and practices lead one to universal truths and achievable transformation.*

As these principles and truths are understood, and the methodology practiced and incorporated into your life's routine, you will become more whole-brained, intuitive, and empowered. You will be less reactive and more responsive. Less resistant and more resonant. Less subjective and more objective. Less mind-directed and more soul-directed. Less fearful and more loving. Sometimes, less is more.

The Inner Sound

The intention I hold in the creation of this book is to assist, guide, and inspire you to look deeper within yourself to recognize and appreciate the wondrous vibrational energy of sound, light, love, and Spirit that resonates within every one of us. It is my sincere hope that you enjoy the ideas, thoughts, feelings, experiences, and exercises shared in the pages to follow. I encourage and support you in utilizing whatever you find to be resonant and useful for your life's repertoire of soul songs, truth tones, life colors—and in "owning your toning."

Keep in mind, however, that for the total healing of body, mind, and Spirit—along with the liberation of the soul—we must learn to be an open conduit for the transformative "inner sound," the Infinite Overtone. As you read further, listen to your body, listen to your heart, listen to your intuition, listen to your soul, listen to your sound, listen to the silence, listen...

(((((2)))))

A Being of Sound Body

Sound is the source of all manifestation....
The knower of the mystery of sound knows
the mystery of the whole universe....

—Hazrat Inayat Khan

Your entire body is made of sound. In fact, everything is made of sound: your clothes, glasses you may be wearing, the book you are holding, whatever you are sitting on, the floor beneath you, the house in which you live, the streets and sidewalks, flowers and trees, the Earth—everything! The whole universe is composed of sound. This principle is now understood by modern scientists, as it has been known by ancient masters for ages.

If you doubt this universal principle, consider the following: Through current scientific technology and new physics research, science has discovered and shown that all matter consists of vibrating waveforms of energy. And though it may not be audible to the human ear, sound is emitted from these waveforms. If you focus on tiny bits of subatomic matter you find they are not material at all, but rather mere vibrations of energy that have taken on the appearance of solidity.

We can measure vibrations by finding their "frequency," or how frequently they vibrate. This is measured in waves or cycles per second called *hertz* (notated as Hz, and named after German physicist Heinrich Hertz, the discoverer of electromagnetic waves), which is the unit for frequency. Energy, sound, frequency, and vibration are merely different aspects of the same principle.

Frequencies of sound also determine the density of matter. Your teeth and bones—the most solid-seeming matter of the body—are composed of energy vibrating at very slow and low frequencies, so they have the most physical density. Your skin, muscles, organs, and other body tissues are vibrating at faster and higher frequency rates, so they have less density.

Then there are the blood and fluids of the body, which vibrate at much faster and higher frequencies, and in turn have much less density. All of this illustrates that your body is literally a human symphony of sound!

As a youngster in elementary school, I can clearly recall the teacher stating, "Much like our planet Earth, our bodies are primarily made of water and consist of approximately 70 percent water and 30 percent solids." I was intrigued with this interesting scientific data. But, as is the case with much in life, I learned after a time that this information was true only from a limited perspective. From a broader, more holistic perspective I discovered that there really are no "solids." Our bodies consist of 100 percent sound.

But is this "body symphony" merely physical? Are we not more than mere "sound sacks" of chemicals? What about our thoughts and feelings? And the soul? If everything is sound and vibration, then these must be as well.

Thoughts and Feelings

Within one vibration are created many vibrations.

—Hazrat Inayat Khan

Just as our so-called physical body does, our thoughts and feelings also consist of sound vibrations, except that these subtle energy waveforms vibrate at faster and higher frequencies. The emotional body, for instance, vibrates at much higher frequencies than the physical, and the mental body at extremely higher rates of frequency than the emotional.

The vibrations of thoughts and feelings are not mere theory. In the 1980s, neuroscientist Candace Pert, Ph.D., made a dramatic breakthrough in discovering that specific brain chemicals called *neuropeptides*—or "chemicals of emotion," as she refers to them—act as couriers between the mind and immune system. Dr. Pert, also the discoverer of endorphins, determined that thoughts not only produce molecules in the brain, but also throughout the body, meaning that the immune system is directly affected by thoughts.

If you want to see what your thoughts were like yesterday, look at your body today. If you want to see what your body will be like tomorrow, look at your thoughts today.

—Indian proverb

Pert has since postulated that our bodies are teeming with our thoughts and emotions, and the mind is actually re-created and evolving on an on-going basis by the interaction of these brain chemicals and receptors. She stresses that the mind and body are not simply linked biologically, but are totally inseparable.

Pert's work has also shown that our gut feelings and intuition are not merely random reactions or illusions, but actual biological realities.

These conclusions are consistent with a growing belief in the healing community that one's attitude and state of mind shape and create the overall health of the body. From a quantum mechanics perspective we can view the mind-body as a silent flow of creative intelligence manifesting in our physical reality. In this context, Deepak Chopra, M.D., in *Perfect Health* states, "The secret of life at this level is that anything in your body can be changed with the flick of intention."

Higher Frequencies

Sound frequencies not only determine the density of matter, but its form as well. The form of a bone or tooth is very defined, whereas the higher frequencies of a muscle or body tissue may be less defined and more malleable. And the still higher frequencies of body fluids such as blood are even less defined in form. Picture blood (or any other liquid) spilling on the floor, and you'll see it never repeats the same shape or pattern. It is amorphous and far less defined in form than the previous examples.

This analogy also gives us an insight into the metaphysical, in that our mental and emotional bodies are vibrating at such high frequencies they function through subtle-energy forms and dimensions. The speed of these frequencies therefore alters our perceptions of time and space as well, when we operate in these modes of awareness.

A human being is part of the whole, called by us "Universe," a part limited in time and space.

> *He experiences himself, his thoughts and feelings as something separated from the rest—a kind of optical delusion of consciousness.*

—Albert Einstein

From a spiritual or metaphysical perspective, the emotional body may be seen in its most complete aspect as the ***astral body***, or the "seat of the emotions." The mental body can be viewed from a similar perspective as the *causal body*, or the seat of higher thought and creativity. However, the spirit or *soul body* vibrates at such incredibly high rates of frequency that they exceed those of the causal body—and all other bodies—extending even beyond time and space. The soul is actually an infinite frequency! And the Sacred Sound Current or Inner Overtone is the real "seat of the soul."

> *The soul is actually an infinite frequency! And the Sacred Sound Current or Inner Overtone is the real "seat of the soul."*

Once we truly experience the infinite vibrations of the Inner Overtone, we begin to realize the eternal nature of the spirit. These spiritual frequencies are impossible for the finite mind to fully comprehend because the dimensions within which these vibrations function are formless, unlimited, and infinite. We can, however, have this blissful and divine experience through the multidimensional frequencies of the soul.

A Question of Consciousness

It now appears that the rates of frequency in the body not only determine the vibrational state of matter, but also reflect the level of one's consciousness. Or, does the level of consciousness determine the frequency and vibrational state of the body?

As you continue this reading journey through the wondrous worlds of the soul, sound, frequency, and vibration, you will begin to understand the significance of this and other related questions. You will also discover secrets to spiritual awareness, healing sounds, and the vibrational power of overtoning.

(((((3)))))

Sound Therapy

All pain and disease are self-created dissonances that assist us in hearing the harmony of the soul.

—Wayne Perry

For decades, sound researchers have explored, tested, developed, and used an assortment of various sound machines, tone generators, and electronic devices to improve health and sustain wellness. Some of these include Rife generators, Tesla coils, radionics machines, frequency modulators, quartz generators, ultrasound, brain wave synchronizers, and self-management auditory devices.

One of the first pioneers in sound research, as well as one of its most controversial figures, is inventor and scientist Royal Raymond Rife. Dr. Rife is probably best known for his invention of an extraordinary microscope that is able to view living cells at 100,000 magnification. While observing the internal activity of human cells, he then developed a frequency generator that, combined with a Ray-O-Vac tube, charged cells with various frequencies.

Beginning in the early 1920s, Rife—according to "The Cancer Cure That Worked," an article by Barry Lynes—discovered a process of killing bacteria by using select frequencies very similar to ultrasonic cleaning. Based on his belief that every diseased organism had its own vibratory signature, Rife and his associates developed the Rife generator, an electronic device used to generate the specific frequencies necessary to destroy the individual microorganisms responsible for cancer and other catastrophic diseases. He eventually found a frequency that would explode and remove diseased cells. With this unique methodology, Rife also found that the cancer cells could be destroyed without damage to the rest of the body.

Although many in the medical community accepted and supported Rife's sound therapies, his unorthodox theories and scientific work upset the ruling powers within this industry. Rife's work was officially stopped, and further research was forced underground.

Since his death in 1971, Rife's bioelectric medical research has gradually become more recognized and accepted by research scientists. Although not officially sanctioned by the medical establishment, to this day Rife-based technology and frequency generators are being explored and reportedly used with success in various sound therapies, including oncology.

Sound Machines

One of the difficulties associated with therapeutic sound machines is that claims of remarkable healing results are difficult to substantiate. There is also concern about the potential dangers inherent with some types of machines, or with their incorrect operation.

> *Just as it does from natural, living, organic, and healthy foods, the body may benefit most from natural sounds for essential "vibrational nutrients."*

For example, receiving a sound treatment with frequencies that are excessive in your signature frequency pattern may push you more out of balance, or exacerbate an existing health concern. This brings up the issue of having to rely on a machine, or the skills and experience of the sound practitioner operating it. You may, of course, educate yourself regarding the operation of sound machines and use them for yourself. However, this could prove to be time-consuming and costly.

It should also be noted that certain people are very "sound-sensitive." When these individuals are exposed to electronic frequencies—"artificial" sound—they often have negative reactions, such as tension, nausea, dizziness, discomfort, and sometimes pain. These symptoms may occur even when receiving targeted sound frequencies that are determined to be deficient and needed by the individual.

Natural Sounds

Bio-acoustic (life sounds) studies have indicated that the likelihood of adverse reactions to sound are greatly reduced by the therapeutic use of organic or natural sound. These types of sounds would include those created by naturally vibrating sources, such as acoustic musical instruments, chimes and bells, crystal bowls, tuning forks, and the voice.

Just as it does from natural, living, organic, and healthy foods, the body may benefit most from natural sounds for essential "vibrational nutrients." They are also the safest sounds, as there have been reports from those sensitive to sound who claim to have adverse reactions to electronically produced or unnatural sounds.

In all the years that I have worked with healing sounds, I know of no circumstance in which listening to the non-amplified, natural overtones and harmonics of an acoustic instrument or the human voice has had any negative effects. The only complaints I have ever encountered have been in regard to either too high a volume, or an unconscious fear or resistance on the part of the listener. These concerns may be easily resolved with a little awareness of sound healing principles (or simply lowering the volume).

The Ear

Although the whole body is a natural receiver for sound frequencies, medical science now informs us that the ear supplies 80 to 90 percent of the bioelectrical energy entering the brain through the five sensory organs. The ear is the first sensory organ to begin functioning—from the eighth week of life in the mother's womb—and by 18 weeks after conception, it has developed to its full size and hearing capacity. Because the ear plays such an active role in affecting the most important areas of the brain, some scientific experts have postulated that the ear controls the entire maturation of the brain.

One such expert is the late French physician, Alfred Tomatis, M.D., renowned for his revolutionary research and clinical work with hearing and sound therapy. Using a device he invented called the Electronic Ear, Dr. Tomatis developed a "Sonic Rebirth" process by which he would assist patients through their earliest developmental periods.

Tomatis used this device to stimulate the muscles of the inner ear and nourish the brain with "charging sounds" rich in high frequencies, and thus re-create the prenatal environment. This procedure would simulate for the individual the journey from the uterus through birth and into early childhood based on how, when, and what one hears. Facilitated by the use of electronically filtered recordings of the mother's voice and musical compositions by Mozart, subjects would reawaken to an earlier consciousness that was psychologically and physically healing.

Modern Technology

Nowadays, a growing number of new sound modalities combine the use of natural sounds with the latest advancements in modern technology. The results of this have given birth to various sound machines, computer programs, tone boxes, and other sonically manageable devices, designed for either diagnostic or therapeutic purposes.

Some of these technologies attempt to create personalized therapeutic frequencies by altering, distorting, or manipulating the sound or pitch of a natural sound, such as the voice. Often used in association with recordings, brainwave entrainment, sympathetic resonance, music, and meditation, this area of sound therapy is rapidly progressing.

Dr. Jeffrey D. Thompson, founder of the Center for Neuroacoustic Research, developed a healing system using recordings of an individual's voice, and playing them through speakers in a specially designed chiropractic table. This system, which he calls Bio-Tuning, uses the sounds in the voice to facilitate self-healing. Dr. Thompson says on his Website, "Only your own vocal cords can produce the unique set of harmonics and overtones which are characteristic of your personal, unique voice-print pattern—a pattern highly recognizable to the part of your biological system which designed and grew your body out of two cells in the first place. This part of the unconscious mind designed the vocal cords themselves and deeply recognizes the unique frequency pattern of sound that they produce."

You may also use your voice to tone along with recordings of your own vocal pattern. Thompson goes on to say, "Your Fundamental Voice-Tone is like your Personal Mantra. The Mantra wasn't just the Sanskrit sound that one used in meditation, but the chanting of one's own special tone, which resonated one's consciousness with one's own vocal cords singing into one's own 'bio-mass' to the root of consciousness." I agree with Dr. Thompson that the imbalances one may experience physically, emotionally, or mentally are external projections of the only real imbalance that can exist—in consciousness itself.

Sound Study

In 1993, as a result of exploring available sound research—and due to my concern about the potential ill effects of electronic sounds mentioned earlier—I decided to abandon my experimentation with sound machines and began using the natural sound frequencies of the voice exclusively in my sound therapy practice. One of the most revealing and inspiring sound studies that contributed greatly to this decision was conducted by some bio-acoustic researchers in the late 1980s, examining the body's responses to various types of sounds. The means of determining these responses was the evaluation of brainwaves and fluctuations in blood pressure.

The sources of sound generation used in the study included a variety of tone generators, sound machines, electronic devices, recorded sounds, musical instruments, and the human voice. The study revealed that when one's personal notes are sounded, of all the sounds tested, those created by the naturally present overtones and harmonics of the human voice are the most supportive and beneficial to the body. A distant second place in this study went to the non-amplified sounds of acoustic musical instruments, with the

> *Sounds created by the naturally present overtones and harmonics of the human voice are the most supportive and beneficial to the body.*

third in effectiveness being an electronically based auditory device designed to mimic the frequency wave patterns of the human voice. The conclusion of the study: Our own voice is our greatest healing sound.

(((((4)))))

Sound Hearing

There are two ways of spreading vibrations: to be the sound, or to be its echo.

—Wayne Perry

To better understand the relationship between sound and the body, it may be helpful to first explore the way we hear sound vibrations. Many of the various sounds, frequencies, and vibrations of the world—as well as the sounds of the "inner worlds"—are indeed inaudible to us, as they are outside the hearing bandwidth of the human ear. Although we may not hear them, these sounds still affect us. This brings to mind the ancient Buddhist koan, which asks, "If a tree falls in the forest and no one is there to hear it, does it make a sound?" We'll explore some of these metaphysical questions, and "unheard" sounds, later. In the meantime, let's look at the human ear and the value in what we can hear.

The anatomy of the human ear allows humans to hear frequency ranges between 16 and 18,000 Hz. The upper and lower boundaries of this bandwidth may be difficult to hear, but many people can hear these frequencies just fine. After approximately 20 years of age, however, most people lose some of their upper range, whereas those younger than 20 usually have the full range of hearing available. The typical human ear can best detect frequencies between 200 and 2,000 Hz. The ear is designed to be most sensitive to these frequencies, although humans usually hear the other sections of the human bandwidth as well.

Animals

Most of us are aware that dogs can hear sounds that we can't. This is why we cannot hear high-pitched dog whistles. What you may not be aware of, however, is that dogs have twice the hearing range/bandwidth of humans, and cats can hear much higher frequencies than dogs! A dog's hearing range starts at a low end, similar to humans. Their upper end range is 40,000 Hz, whereas cats can hear up to 60,000 Hz. However, cats do not

> *Dolphins and Orcas have the ability to hear the highest frequencies—about 10 times higher than that of humans!*

have the same low-range hearing capabilities as dogs or humans. The lowest sound that cats can hear is about 80 Hz.

Bats have a much greater bandwidth of hearing, with the low end at a deep 10 Hz, and a high end at 110,000 Hz. Although they may not hear sounds as low as bats do, dolphins and Orcas have the greatest bandwidth and ability to hear the highest frequencies—about 10 times higher than that of humans! The dolphin's hearing ranges anywhere from 110 to around 200,000 Hz.

Ultrasonic Sounds

Sounds with frequencies above the 18,000 Hz human bandwidth of hearing are referred to as *ultrasonic* sounds. Sounds that resonate below the 16 Hz range of human hearing are called *infrasonic* or *subsonic* sounds. Although these types of sounds—above and below the human hearing range—may not be heard by people, they definitely exist in the environment. Animals are quite sensitive to ultrasonic sounds. Bats, for example, use ultrasonic sounds as a tool for navigation and hunting. Dolphins use ultrasonic frequencies to communicate with each other.

> *The low-frequency sound waves emitted from a bridge may not be audible to the human ear, but it is speculated that the waves may affect the heart.*

Infrasonic Sounds

Slow-vibrating objects—such as buildings or bridges—produce infrasonic sounds with frequencies of less than 20 Hz. Understanding some fundamentals regarding these unheard sounds has added significance in a therapeutic context. There have been studies suggesting that the "silent sound pollution" of vibrating infrasonic frequencies generated by bridges may encourage heart dysrhythmia in people living near them. The low-frequency sound waves emitted from a bridge may not be audible to the human ear, but it is speculated (though not proven) that the waves may affect the heart.

A few more interesting sound facts: Elephants are known to make sounds as low as 12 Hz, and nuclear explosions can produce infrasonic sounds as low as 0.01 Hz. Further, scientists have discovered—quite by accident, using sound sensors that detect infrasonic sound frequencies—that the spinning vortex of a tornado produces sounds that are a few hertz below the human hearing range. Because these infrasonic sound waves can be detected by sound sensor machines up to 100 miles away, this may help increase the warning time for tornado strikes.

Ultrasound

We mustn't confuse ultrasonic sound with **ultrasound**. Ultrasound is a method of looking inside a person's body to examine tissue and liquid-based organs without physically entering the body. It is sometimes used instead of X-rays, for it does not employ radiation and is safer for the person being examined. Ultrasound is commonly used by obstetricians to examine the progress of a woman's fetus during pregnancy.

This technology is also used to observe the status of different organs and systems in the body, such as the nervous, circulatory, urinary, and reproductive systems. Ultrasound methods direct high-frequency sound into particular areas of the body and measure the time it takes for the sound waves to reflect back to the transmitting machine. By analyzing the pattern of reflections received, a computer can create a visual representation on a monitor.

Therapeutic success has also been achieved in patients suffering from ailments such as kidney stones by directing these high-frequency sounds into the kidneys to shatter the stones. Research in the therapeutic uses of ultrasound continues to develop.

Ear "Rings"

Although it is difficult to substantiate information on all the deleterious effects of ultrasonic and infrasonic sounds, the effects of some types of sound and noise pollution may more easily be viewed as dangerous. For instance, have you ever experienced the discomfort of "ringing in the ears" after leaving a loud rock concert? The ringing sound is a result of the destruction of the cilia (little hairs of varying lengths inside the cochlea of the ear) by high-volume sounds. The cilia resonate when a sound reaches the hair's natural frequency. If a sound is extremely loud and goes on for some period of time, it can damage the cilia and even kill it. The ringing sensation is actually the cilia dying! Usually the ringing disappears, but permanent damage has already been done. The hair cells can never grow back.

The effects of such hearing loss may take repeated exposure over the years to become apparent, but can become devastating nonetheless. For some, the results can be tinnitus, a severe roaring or ringing in the ears that may require surgery. As a sound therapist over the years I have assisted various clients—particularly drummers, electric guitarists, and other musicians—in getting relief from this debilitating condition.

Intensity and Protection

If you have had any type of similar experience of ringing ears or other discomfort, here are two easy and immediate ways to protect yourself. First, increase the distance between your ears and the speakers or source of the loud sounds. The farther you are from the sound source, the lower the intensity of the sound. By simply doubling the distance, the intensity becomes one-fourth of what it was originally. Second, to protect yourself from hearing damage, deaden or dampen the sound waves entering the ear by wearing earplugs. Be sure to use earplugs with an adequate defense against high-decibel sound. For example, swimming-type earplugs are designed to keep water out of the ears but may not shield sound adequately. A set of sleeping-type earplugs in the 25-decibel range should be sufficient for most situations.

Decibels

The decibel (dB), is the internationally adopted unit for the relative intensity of sound. The intensity is relative because the measurement compares a loudness level to a reference level, usually the threshold of human hearing. The hearing threshold is usually referenced at 0, or one decibel.

The following on page 36 shows examples of a typical sound environment and the relative intensity of various sounds compared to the threshold of hearing.

In studying these examples of environmental sounds and their corresponding intensity (decibels), it is important to understand an additional factor. The decibel scale is a logarithmic scale: For every 10 dBs, the loudness of a sound is increased by a factor of 10. For example, a relative intensity change of 50 dBs to 60 dBs means the sound will be 10 times louder than it was at 50 dBs. A change of 50 dBs to 70 dBs would mean the new sound would be 100 times as loud.

Sound Type	Decibels (dBs)	Sound Type	Decibels (dBs)
Hearing Threshold	0	Lawnmower	100
Breathing	10	Rock Concert	110
Whisper	30	Pain Threshold	120
Normal Speaking	50	Jet Engine	130
Automobile Traffic	70	Rocket Launch	140
Factory	90	Hearing Loss	150

Another vital point on sound intensity: The threshold of pain for humans depends upon the individual, but typically ranges between 120 dBs and 130 dBs. For example, if you are in close proximity to jackhammers, jet engines, or rocket launches, or present at an extremely loud rock concert, you may experience such pain. Keep in mind that sound intensity exceeding 150 dBs can result in loss of hearing. Interestingly, recent studies have shown that the animal with the loudest sound on earth is the blue whale at 188 dBs!

Several years ago, an interesting yet somewhat frightening experiment was conducted by a small group of scientists using high-intensity sound with a "sound cannon." Thirty thousand acoustic watts were generated and broadcast through a modulator and a large 10-foot horn into a sealed acoustic chamber containing a solid brick wall. The scientists wanted to determine the effects of high-intensity sound on the wall. The sound vibrations were trapped and intensified by the enclosed space to enable the sound to crumble and shatter the wall. If a human being were exposed to sound at the test volume, it would not only cause permanent hearing loss, but internal organs would also be damaged, and the exposure could even prove deadly!

Could the Israelites have created enough sound volume to cause the walls of Jericho to vibrate and crumble? Some believe this biblical account implies knowledge of the properties of sound that could not have been known by the people of that era. Perhaps they were divinely guided to use sound as a means of achieving their goal.

Ear to Voice

Another result of sound research reveals to us that all the sounds we make with the voice are totally dependent on and reflect all the sounds we hear with the ears. In other words, if you can hear a sound, unless you are mute, you can potentially make that sound. Although some sounds may be above or below your vocal range, if you can hear them, you can approximate the tone or timbre of the sound. Conversely, if you can't hear a sound, you have no reference for making the sound.

> *All the sounds we make with the voice are totally dependent on and reflect all the sounds we hear with the ears.*

This principle illustrates why those who are deaf (since birth) have difficulty enunciating words and speaking. We need to hear the sounds of the words, syllables, and vowels in order to properly speak them. (This is why it's difficult to get a French or German accent exactly right if it isn't your primary language or you aren't frequently around others who speak these languages.) The hearing impaired, consequently, rely more on their senses of sight and touch for accessing information, yet they may be very sensitive to feeling sound vibrations.

Accents

This also illustrates why people who live in various areas of the United States have different regional accents. For example, those living in the South and southeastern part of the country speak with a "Southern drawl," quite different from those living in the southwest or northern regions. The New York accent of Easterners greatly differs from the regional accents of Midwesterners or Texans.

These differences in speaking accents are fairly obvious, but there are also subtler speech differences, less noticeable, between those living in closer proximity—for instance, between people living in Massachusetts and New York, or between those in Illinois and Minnesota, or Oregon and Arizona. Similar examples of vocal accents can be observed in different languages and dialects within various regions and countries throughout the world.

Environments

We unconsciously take on the speech patterns, inflections, and accents of people in our environment. Though this may change if we move to a new state or country, the longer we live in a particular area, the more we tend to retain the vocal patterns of that area. Living in California since 1985, I've lost much of my Midwestern accent. However, whenever I spend time visiting family and friends in my former hometown of Chicago, I frequently find my voice beginning to take on the speech characteristics of that area.

Many are not even aware of their regional accents until moving to a different environment, or having it pointed out to them. Unless one is professionally involved in public speaking, teaching, or acting, a foreign or regional accent may not be of concern. But by learning improved listening skills and proper vocal exercises, one can easily change these vocal habits, if desired. There are also many voice and diction coaches who commonly work with those who wish to free themselves from deeply ingrained or strong accents.

Remembering

In the next few chapters, you will discover the value of listening to the sound in others' voices, as well as the words. You can learn volumes about someone through the sound of their voice. You will discover the "secrets" in the sound of your own voice. You'll also learn even more about yourself through voicing your sound, and ultimately your soul. This will enable you to more consciously create and affect your "sound" environment. This is important from an auditory perspective, and vital from a vibrational one. You live in a world of sound. You indeed are sound—"a being of sound body." Your voice is the expression of that sound. Remember who you really are.

P ART II

Toning and the Voice

The voice is an expression of our character, our very soul, and everything we are. Therefore, it has great power to influence our lives and the lives of others

(((((5)))))

The Vocal Mechanism

The voice is not only indicative of man's character,
but it is the expression of his spirit.

—Hazrat Inayat Khan

No instrument ever invented has the facility to create and manipulate sounds as the human voice does. Through use of the unique and comprehensive vocal mechanism, we can speak, shout, whisper, laugh, cry, moan, tone, hum, and sing—all with natural ease. Our facility for vocal expression has developed over thousands of years, along with the evolution of the brain and intellectual faculties.

As we look back through prehistoric time and our evolutionary process, we discover that vocal expression and primitive communication, at some point, began to dramatically influence quality of life. Evidence shows that chanting may have preceded speaking, and, even before then, various sounding and toning led to chanting and singing. Human speech wasn't significantly developed until the fourth Ice Age, some 70,000 years ago. From that point on, with the explosion of human population and the challenges of survival, speech became an absolute necessity and made great leaps forward.

Stimulated by social evolution and cultural sophistication, speech was further developed and writing was birthed. More than 3,000 languages were created, and modern humankind—the top of creation—stepped forth to claim its dominion over the world. Fighting our way to the top of the animal kingdom has been a long and extraordinary journey that has surely been made successful by the development of the human voice.

One of the most important topics explored in this book is the optimal methods through which the voice may be understood, used, controlled, developed, and freed. In this methodology, we learn to open and release the voice for enhancing communication skills, social confidence, personal power, physical and emotional health, and spiritual awareness.

Although there are three principal ways in which we express the voice—speaking, singing or chanting, and toning—we will primarily focus on the latter. Before we discuss various techniques, practices, and benefits associated with toning, it will be helpful to first examine the mechanics of the voice.

Basic Functions

The process of producing vocal sounds is called **phonation**. Good phonation occurs when we properly use the vocal instrument. Before exploring the techniques for maximizing the full potential of the human voice, let's examine its basic functions.

The vocal mechanism is an extraordinary instrument that relies on the coordination of several separate components that drive these functions: the lungs, diaphragm, larynx, vocal cords, pharynx, throat, mouth, tongue, and nasal cavities. When all of these components are synchronized and used properly, a magically resonant vocal expression can be achieved.

The four basic functions of the voice and its components are:

1. Generation.
2. Vibration.
3. Resonation.
4. Articulation.

1. Generation

As the vocal foundation, power is generated through the voice by the lungs and diaphragm. The airstream is then concentrated and channeled by the trachea and bronchi and sent to the larynx. When inflated as we breathe, the lungs act as a pair of bellows, providing the air pressure necessary to vibrate the vocal cords. This produces the power for the voice to sound. The trachea is also known as the windpipe—hence the commonly used phrase "he (or she) has a great set of pipes!"

Vocalizing requires the delicate orchestration of almost 60 muscles just to sing the notes: "do, re, me." But don't be intimidated: Most of these muscles are used involuntarily and unconsciously. However, the single most important muscle in sounding the voice is the diaphragm. It is a powerful sheet of muscular tissue that separates the chest cavity from the abdominal cavity. Inhalation takes place as we contract and lower the diaphragm, enlarging the chest cavity, thereby pulling air into our lungs. To exhale, we simply relax the diaphragm; thus the chest cavity shrinks and presses air out from our lungs.

2. Vibration

As air is exhaled from the lungs it passes through the larynx or voice box. The larynx sets up voice vibrations, similar to a tuning fork. It is a tube-shaped mechanism in the throat that consists of many delicate muscles and cartilages, and it houses and protects the vocal cords. Although the larynx is the organ that transforms the airstream into specific vibrational patterns, the actual sound is produced by the vocal cords.

These "cords" should more correctly be referred to as vocal folds, for they are not cordlike at all. They are actually two protuberances of mucous membrane that line the larynx wall. These vocal folds are connected across the windpipe in an elastic, V-shaped configuration. They are fixed together at the front of the throat, with the other end of each fold connected separately to two mobile cartilages at the back of the throat. Muscles move the cartilage, pulling the vocal folds together, allowing them to vibrate in the airstream from the lungs. When we strain or overuse the voice, these folds have difficulty pulling together, with the results being hoarseness or, even worse, laryngitis.

Directly above the vocal folds are two "false folds." These false folds are not used for vocal sounding, but they, along with the vocal folds, help to protect the lungs from inhaling debris. When the false folds are tightly drawn together, they help us hold our breath. Our lungs could actually collapse were it not for the fact that we involuntarily hold our breath when we exert ourselves physically. We should be grateful for these little wonders of nature!

Another one of nature's little gifts is the epiglottis. Located at the base of the tongue, at the top of the windpipe, this thin cartilaginous flap of tissue folds back and protects the glottis during swallowing. Thus, it helps prevent food and liquid from entering the larynx and choking off our air supply. The elongated space between the vocal folds, and the structures that surround this space, is the glottis. The opening and closing of the glottis can manipulate vocal sound with the pressure of breath.

3. Resonation

Just behind the epiglottis lies an elastic chamber referred to as the pharynx. The mouth and pharynx act as resonators for sound. Once the larynx generates a vocal tone, it must be empowered and enhanced by resonation within the pharynx, mouth, and nasal passages, in the same way that the hollow body of a guitar or other stringed instrument amplifies its musical tones. Sound complexity increases, giving the human voice its richness and resonance as the throat and oral and nasal cavities vibrate with vocal overtones. These are the primary areas of resonation and amplification.

Secondary resonators include the chest cavity, skull, bones, and carti-lage. The voice finds its best resonation in hard, conducting surfaces and clearly defined hollows within the body structure. These various conduc-tors and amplifiers resonate an intriguing array of overtones, which make up the timbre and sound color of the voice. Sounds created in the process of resonation may be further developed and enhanced by articulation.

4. Articulation

The primary articulators are the mouth, lips, and tongue, which allow us to mold, shape, and embellish sound. The mouth represents the last point of departure for the voice. Secondary articulators include the glottis, teeth, gums, uvula, and hard and soft palates. All these organic tools are located primarily in the upper third of the vocal apparatus, mostly in what's referred to as the *vocal mask*. This mask is situated where the primary articulators and resonators are (specifically, from the bridge of the nose and nasal cavities, down to the jaw and upper throat area).

When we place and project the voice forward, from the mask rather than from the lower throat, we put much less stress on the voice and vocal cords. This results in enhanced vocal quality, range and power. By learn-ing to speak, sing, and tone through the vocal mask, the voice opens and becomes more flexible, resonant, and articulate.

Understanding and developing skills in the articulation process gives us the freedom to create greater vocal expression, including enhanced aesthetic appeal and vibrational healing benefits.

≈

A few other aspects of the voice warrant discussion here.

Pitch

Vocal pitch is determined by the frequency, speed, or number of cycles per second with which the vocal folds vibrate to produce the tone of the voice. The pitch could also be viewed as the determination of a musical sound, proceeding from low to high in the tonal scale. Whereas the exact pitch within a given range is determined by such variables as tension of the vocal folds and the air pressure, the range of the voice is dependent upon the size of the larynx as related to age, sex, body type, and vocal development.

We may change the pitch of our vocal sounds by manipulating a comprehensive array of muscles in and around the larynx. In a whisper, for instance, we pull the vocal folds together only slightly, and, for singing or toning, the folds are drawn in completely. The thinner the vocal folds, the faster the vibrations and the higher the pitch of the tone. The vocal folds operate under the same principle as stretching the neck of an inflated balloon while slowly releasing its air to make a squealing sound. Another example is the way in which a guitarist may raise the pitch of a guitar string to a higher note by stretching or tightening it at the tuning peg.

To increase the volume of the voice, we simply raise the speed and pressure of air coming out from our lungs. Keep in mind, however, that breathing and vocalizing are not simply manipulations of muscles by nerves. They involve states of awareness on many levels. This is why our voices reflect our inner energies and personal vibrations.

Special note: During sexual excitement and lovemaking, the mucous membrane of the larynx undergoes physical changes that cause the voice to become deeper and huskier. Therefore the sexiness of that low, husky whisper is rooted in biology. Universally admired and simulated by men and women alike, the soft murmurs of singers and movie stars harkens back to imitations of this sexy voice!

Vocal Registers

There are three basic vocal registers: the chest voice, the mid-voice, and the head voice (also referred to as the falsetto). This reflects the elementary fact that low notes are felt mostly in the chest, and high notes are usually felt in the head. However, another register may be used to produce extremely high notes. It is referred to as the *whistle register*, and is called so because the vocal folds are tightened to a razor-sharp edge, allowing a small, elliptical hole to form between them. In this register the folds do not even vibrate. The vocal sound literally whistles through this hole.

In addition to its use as an upper register, stylistic singing technique, this high whistle may be developed in creating multiple tones or overtones with the voice. (These toning methods will be addressed in detail in Chapter 12.)

Natural Range and Pitch

For the serious student of the voice, it is important to recognize and use your natural range and pitch. In the average individual, the natural speaking range is between one and one and a half octaves. The natural singing range may expand to more octaves due to the generation of more vocal power.

Unfortunately, most of us adopt unnatural voices—either consciously, unconsciously, or both—unaware of our natural frequency. We often copy and imitate others' speaking or singing voices that we find appealing. For evidence of this, just turn on the TV or radio for an example of the redundancy in the voices of most popular singers and announcers. We hear the same vocal styles copied over and over again.

By projecting our voice through the resonators mentioned earlier, we must find the natural pitch frequency and octave appropriate for our vocal range. A piano, a guitar, a set of tuning forks, or even a pitch pipe may be used to help you discover your natural vocal range. In relation to middle C, simply find the lowest and highest notes you can sing without strain or total loss of quality. This is your singing range. Your natural speaking range will be within the octave around the midpoint of your voice.

During vocal projection, unnatural forcing of the voice may "feed back" to the vocal folds, negating accurate control of pitch, tone, and volume. Never force your sound or strain your voice. To prevent this needless, potentially damaging, and often common habit of "vocal aggression," it is necessary that you use breath and vocal relaxation methods to release the tensions accumulated in the voice by physical and emotional stress. (Refer to Chapter 7 and Chapter 8.)

Don't try to sound the way someone else does. Only you have the perfect voice for the true expression of your heart and soul.

The importance of using and developing your natural range and pitch cannot be overemphasized, as any other pitch that is unnatural for you will strain the vocal mechanisms. With proper use, the natural pitch will develop, become more flexible, and expand naturally in range. Don't try to sound the way someone else does. Only you have the perfect voice for the true expression of your heart and soul. Own your tone.

After exploring your vocal mechanism and establishing a sound foundation of voice awareness, allow your tones to flow naturally through your body. Remember that your whole body is your instrument. Let the "sound of your soul" play your instrument. Familiarize yourself with the vast array of frequencies in your body-instrument. You will not only develop enhanced vocal capabilities, but also deepen your awareness of the vibrational role of your soul.

> *Your whole body is your instrument. Familiarize yourself with the vast array of frequencies in your body-instrument.*

Natural Range and Pitch Exercise

Read aloud a paragraph from a book you enjoy. Elongate the vowels and connect the words as if singing them. Repeat the paragraph while making up a simple melody, then sing the words with the melody. Keep singing the paragraph while adjusting your volume and pitch (high and low voice). Without straining your voice with too loud a volume or erratic shifts in pitch, repeat your melody to the words. This is your natural pitch.

≈

(((((6)))))

The Human Voice: The Ultimate Healing Instrument

*The voice has all the magnetism which an instrument
lacks; for voice is nature's ideal instrument, upon which
all other instruments of the world are modeled.*

—Hazrat Inayat Khan

The human voice can be used to increase self-awareness and to heal yourself. The voice releases power in the direction of our thoughts and feelings, thereby sending vibrations throughout the body. As we learn to control and direct these vocal vibrations appropriately, we can restore harmony and balance to particular body systems. This vocal practice is the essence of toning, and shifts the vibrational pattern of the body to its perfect electromagnetic field.

Toning

The most multidimensional aspect of the voice is toning. This is, in part, because toning does not rely as strongly on the left-brain, structural components necessary for speaking, singing, and chanting. Toning is a more right-brain vocal method in that it is rooted less in traditional vocalizing or musical foundations and more in the spontaneous and intuitive expression of feelings. However, when some toning techniques are incorporated— without inhibiting creative expression—toning can be enhanced and used in a very powerful and conscious "whole brain" manner.

We could view toning from two perspectives: conscious or unconscious. With unconscious toning, for example, we might moan, groan, sigh, or hum to naturally relieve tension or stress. During conscious toning, however, we hold a specific intent to achieve a desired result with the sound produced. This practice is much more powerful and effective in achieving and sustaining mind-body wellness, and will be addressed throughout this book.

48

The basis of toning is the use of elongated tones and sustained sounds—primarily, but not limited to, vowels—to change, release, or transform vibrational energy. Toning may also represent a spontaneous vocal expression that reflects and accompanies an expansion of human awareness and/or spiritual development.

Toning could be further defined as a vocal practice designed to use sound for the release or transformation of energy blockages in the body. It's a natural and organic vibrational healing tool—available to anyone with a voice—for harmonizing and balancing energy fields.

As we develop skills with toning, we can learn to immediately relax tension, release stress and pain, clear and balance the chakras, regenerate and re-create body systems, restore harmony and homeostasis to the body, and advance awareness in higher consciousness. If this "sounds" too good to be true, I invite you to explore the world of toning and "The Human Voice: The Ultimate Healing Instrument."

Before we examine the various principles and exercises associated with the toning process, it is necessary to create a solid foundation upon which you can build a strong and enduring vocal structure. The following information and methodology will assist you in this endeavor.

Vocal Quality

Learning the characteristics that determine vocal quality can be most useful in evaluating and developing the voice. Listening closely to others' voices, and especially recording and listening to your own voice, are the best ways to use this information for vocal development. As you examine the following vocal characteristics and their opposite polarities, you may wish to note where your voice lies and which qualities you wish to enhance and develop:

≈ **Timbre (Tonal Color):** Full, strong, bright, and energetic, or thin, weak, dull, and lifeless.

≈ **Texture:** Resonant, smooth, and clear, or cracking, rough, and raspy.

≈ **Volume:** Well-modulated, appropriate, and easily adaptable, or too soft or loud, inappropriate, and not easily adaptable.

≈ **Enunciation:** Distinct, clearly articulated, and with appropriate emphasis, or slurred, poorly articulated, and with inappropriate emphasis.

≈ **Delivery:** Natural, unforced, relaxed, and open, or strained, forced, constricted, and blocked.

≈ **Flow:** Evenly paced, fully integrated, appropriate dynamics, and good resolution, or erratically paced, words run together, starts or stops abruptly, and trails off.

≈ **Attitude/Spirit:** Enthusiastic yet calm, confident, self-loving, and appealing, or repressed, nervous, fearful, and repelling.

With an ongoing awareness of these characteristics of vocal quality and a clear intention regarding what you want to improve, you will be able to successfully use the upcoming information and exercises to further enhance your voice.

Tuning Your Instrument

In a similar manner to how we would tune a guitar or piano to obtain the purest, most harmonious sound, we must tune our vocal instrument. We do this not just by listening and adjusting our pitch—which is indeed important—but also by being aware of pitch from another perspective: When and why does our pitch rise, lower, or waver while speaking? How aware of it are we when it occurs? And what causes this?

The next related aspect of the voice we need to consider is volume. When and why does our speaking volume unconsciously get louder or softer? How aware are we of this? Does this routinely occur only with particular people and situations, or more frequently and arbitrarily? How quickly and easily can we adjust our volume appropriately?

A third important vocal factor is our meter, or speed of delivery. Can we notice our voice speeding up and running words together, or slowing down with unnecessary stops, starts, and pauses? Does this occur regularly, or only in certain situations? What are those situations? Why does this happen?

Getting to Know Your Voice

When we lose discipline and control of our thoughts and emotions, it is reflected in our voice. This is most evident in the three vocal aspects indicated previously: pitch, volume, and meter. For example, when we are feeling enthusiastic, anxious, angry, or upset, the voice frequently rises in pitch and volume, and may speed up in meter or delivery. When we feel sad, sexual, lonely, or depressed, the voice may lower in pitch and volume, and slow down.

By taking note of what circumstances surround these changes in our voice—and monitoring our thoughts and feelings when they occur—we can increase our vocal awareness and recapture control. The following exercise will assist you in isolating these aspects of the voice and gain greater vocal discipline and integration.

Voice Control Exercise

Talk for five minutes or so about something you've recently done that has importance to you. (This works best if you speak into a recording device.) Play back the recording while focusing attention on any rising or falling of your pitch. Does it sound and feel natural and appropriate? Do you notice any particular thoughts or feelings influencing your pitch? Are you satisfied with your pitch, or do you wish to alter it? Note your responses.

Now put your attention on any shifts in your volume, and ask yourself the same questions. Then focus on your meter or speed of delivery. Are you speaking too slow or fast? Are there any inappropriate rushes or pauses in your speech pattern? Is this impacting proper enunciation? Are you running any words together? Again, notice if you'd like to improve your vocal meter and note your response.

After gaining some awareness of your vocal patterns, try recording and listening back to your voice while talking about a painful or uncomfortable situation that you've experienced, and then listen to it. Again, monitor your speech pattern with regard to pitch, volume, and meter. Notice any differences in your voice from the previous exercise. What aspects of your voice would you like to gain better control over? If you're still not clear, try the process again, discussing and recording any emotionally charged issues—positive or negative, past, present, or future.

≈

Voice Control

Once you are clear about what needs to be "tuned" or improved in your voice, take each aspect individually and work with it. First, develop a natural, unforced pitch. Practice a well-modulated and appropriate volume. And then, pace your speed of delivery for a natural meter and appropriate flow of speech. When you feel confident that you have achieved the necessary technique, re-record your voice and listen for improvement. Fine-tune your voice until satisfied. With a little awareness and practice of these three vocal aspects, you will gain greater voice control.

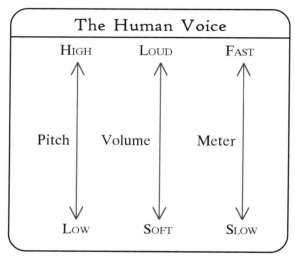

Level 2 pitch, volume, meter

The diagram shown here will assist you in tuning your voice by identifying where your voice falls in terms of pitch, volume, and meter. You may wish to copy or draw the vertical arrows on a separate paper, so that you can mark them with a pen at the points where you feel your voice is located. Re-mark them as you improve your vocal control and quality.

You may also gain much improvement in these aspects of vocal control by practicing with others. These exercises can greatly assist you:

≈ Invite a friend or family member to listen to your voice and give you feedback on pitch, volume, and meter. Examine how it compares with your previous exercises and self-evaluation.

≈ Ask another if he/she will allow you to evaluate his/her voice and vocal aspects. (Give feedback only if he/she requests it.)

≈ Trade off with another and create different voice patterns by changing their aspects. Interpret each other's patterns.

≈ Create a vocal pattern for someone and have him/her create one for you. Listen for understanding and accuracy of interpretation.

≈ Start or join a vocal support group for feedback and discussion.

Changes in voice quality, such as those indicated previously, are directly related to our inner voice as well as the outer voice. They are also vocal indicators of our signature frequency. When we are out of vibrational balance, the pitch, volume, and meter of the voice clearly demonstrates this. When we work from within to establish a holistically integrated voice, or "Whole Voice," we can achieve vibrational balance and resonance. This then becomes obvious in our outer voice, after sound practice and vocal transformation.

Vocal Maturity

Our physical and emotional development is closely related to the sound of our voice. This can be observed (and heard) throughout infancy, adolescence, adulthood, and old age. For example, when adolescents go through puberty, important personal growth and transformation occurs. It is an indication of both physical and emotional growth.

> *Changes in voice quality are directly related to our inner voice as well as the outer voice.*

During this time of maturity, certain vibrational energy centers, or chakras, open and become activated. (See Chapter 10.) An individual is then motivated to develop and assert his or her energies in new ways. Some of these may include: greater independence (first chakra); an increase in hormonal activity and sexual feelings (second chakra); changes in self-consciousness, confidence, willpower, and ego (third chakra); heightened feelings and emotional sensitivity (fourth chakra); greater creativity and vocal expression of thoughts and feelings (fifth chakra); stronger mental activity, intuition, aspirations, and opinions (sixth chakra); spirituality, enlightenment, transcendence, and oneness (seventh chakra). This phenomenon of human growth is all reflected in the voice.

Elements of the Voice

Another perspective for better understanding the vocal instrument may be gained by examining the "voice elements." Vibrational energy may be divided into five elements: Earth, Water, Fire, Air, and Ether. These elements relate and interact to create all life. They are also expressed by the human voice and are stimulated according to the predominant elements present and accessed.

By understanding which elements are primary and secondary in our voice, we can learn how to improve vocal integration, quality, and control. The following descriptions outline how the voice is affected by the five elements.

1. The **Earth Voice** is deep, grounded, solid, and secure in its nature and tonal color. The earth quality is strong, resonant, encouraging, and supportive. The pitch is low. The volume is soft. The speed of meter is slow and measured. This relates to the first chakra.

2. The **Water Voice** is fluid, connected, creative, and emotional in its nature and tonal color. The water quality is smooth, soothing, and intoxicating. The pitch is between the low and mid-voice. The volume is between soft and medium levels. The meter is between slow and medium speeds. This relates to the second chakra.

3. The **Fire Voice** is sharp, distinct, driving, and awakening in nature and tonal color. The fire quality is arousing, enthusiastic, and dramatic. The pitch runs from the middle to high voice. The volume is medium to loud. The meter/speed is medium to fast. This relates to the third chakra.

4. The **Air Voice** is unpredictable, shifting, and expansive in its nature and tonal color. The air quality is light, breathy, and uplifting. The pitch is high. The volume is loud. The meter/speed is fast. This relates to the fourth chakra.

5. The **Etheric Voice (Whole Voice)** is open, free, convincing, harmonious, sacred, and silent in its nature and tonal color. The ether quality is full, resonant, healing, inspiring, and appealing. The pitch is varied, integrated, and complete. The volume is well modulated and comprehensive. The meter/speed is evenly paced and in the present moment. The Etheric Voice reflects the space in sound and the sound of silence. This relates to the fifth chakra, but interacts with all the chakras.

By listening closely to our own voice and the voices of others, we can discover the dominant element that is expressed. Although all the elements are present in the voice, some have a secondary influence, and one or more may even be dormant.

Voice Elements Exercise

As an exercise, record your voice while speaking and then listen to identify elements that may be weak or dormant. You may then use the information previously outlined for practicing the strengthening and integration of those voice elements. Record and monitor yourself from time to time for finer tuning and optimum voice development.

≈

The Whole Voice

Fully exploring and understanding the voice is a wonderful discipline for developing the art of listening and is a key element in self-realization. As we become more aware of our own voices, we begin to hear and intuit the unspoken intentions behind—and within—the voices of others. The way we express ourselves through the voice reflects who we are. The voice gives essential insights into one's complete being. Each accumulated life experience—internal and external—leaves its imprint on our brainwave patterns and vibrational bodies. These patterns then develop and evolve through time and with our individual maturation process. Our voices reflect our "wholeness," or lack thereof—physically, emotionally, mentally, and spiritually.

In *The Book of Sound Therapy*, Olivea Dewhurst-Maddock says, "The voice reflects the mental, emotional and physical condition of a person: it is truly a parable of the soul. In the same way that the soul links the personality of the individual to the spiritual unity of the whole, the voice links the smallest wave or particle of energy to the energy of the Universe." Therefore, the voice is diagnostic as well as therapeutic, and may be easily understood and developed with practice and the assistance of a skilled sound therapist or vibrational healer. (This methodology is addressed in more detail in Chapter 13.)

The sound of your voice reflects your personality and overall state of being. It indicates your own unique personal vibration. The voice also reveals your character and expresses your soul's essence. In his book, *Sacred Sounds: Transformation Through Music & Word*, author Ted Andrews says, "The voice responds instinctively to the energy and condition of the spirit and soul of the individual. It is for this reason that we need to increase awareness of the occult significance of speech."

Sound Feelings Exercise

The human voice is an incredibly powerful yet profoundly sensitive instrument. It has an indelible influence upon the meaning and effect of our words and sounds. The voice is the perfect vehicle for mental and emotional expression.

To experience this vocal phenomenon, try this exercise: Select any vowel sound, let's say "A" ("AY"). Think of a feeling you've once had and take a moment to really feel it. Then tone the "A" sound while imbuing it with that feeling. Notice how it sounds. Now try a different feeling using the same method and vowel sound. As you express the new feeling, notice the difference in the texture of the sound. Is it more aggressive? Tentative? Rough or smooth? Louder or softer? What other differences can you notice?

Continue the exercise by repeating the process using different feelings, but only the "A" sound. Don't repress or edit your sounds. To support your process, here's a partial list of some feelings you can tone with the "A" sound:

Surprise	Confusion	Fun	Envy
Impatience	Scared	Anger	Guilt
Doubt	Release	Joy	Carefree
Boredom	Grief	Hot	Exhaustion
Irritation	Sexual	Cold	Gratitude
Happiness	Skeptical	Fear	Repression
Sadness	Funny	Love	Serenity

Take note of the similarity between the sounds of different feelings. And notice the vast array of feelings that can be conveyed by just one simple sound! If so much can be expressed by just one single vowel sound, imagine how much can be communicated, received, experienced, felt, and learned by multiple sounds.

Our emotions are completely and inextricably connected to the sound of our voice. Therefore, sound reflects all of our thoughts and feelings—not to mention our soul. Think about how many ways we can say the following statement: "I like you a lot." It can be spoken with love, sarcasm, respect, dishonesty, fear, joy, satisfaction, anger, or lust. The volume of the voice, pitch, speed, and word emphasis can alter the meaning as well. Exactly what the sentence means will depend largely upon how it is spoken by the individual, and every individual will express it differently.

To fully experience this principle, speak the sentence, "I like you a lot" several times, consecutively. Shift the accent or emphasis between the various words. For example, "I LIKE you a lot," or "I like YOU a lot." Notice how the meaning changes. Continue the exercise by increasing or decreasing your volume, raising and lowering your pitch, and speeding up and slowing down the words. Think about how different feelings and intentions might affect your vocal expression.

Reading Voice Patterns

We can learn a great deal about an individual by simply listening closely to different aspects of his/her vocal patterns. For example, sadness and depression in a voice results in a slow or trembling articulation—usually accompanied by a very monotone speech pattern. There are often frequent pauses, along with a "trailing off" volume at the end of sentences. Anger is reflected by a rising pitch and over-articulation of certain words or syllables. There is often an increase in meter or speed of vocal delivery, and a flustered mispronunciation of words.

In general, uneven and off-pitch sounds represent imbalances in the third or fifth chakras (see Chapter 10), indicating an unwillingness or inability to address significant personal issues going on. A dull and lifeless voice may be a symptom of low prana or a depletion of life force energy and vitality. Those who are overly talkative or taciturn often have chronic emotional imbalances.

Deeply held fears often reveal themselves in voices that are erratic with radical shifts in volume, pitch, speed, or timbre. Conversely, those whose voices are resonant, well modulated, evenly tempered and metered, and calm, and that overall sound appealing and captivating, are usually imbued with a loving and peaceful heart. This type of individual reflects a balanced and harmonious signature frequency and a "Whole Voice." This fully realized voice emerges only when the inner and outer vibrational energies are developed and integrated.

Note: It is important not to confuse an attractive or pleasant-sounding voice with the Whole Voice. Any radio announcer, game show host, or voice coach may be trained to speak properly and sound "aesthetically pleasing." This type of voice can be misleading. Though it may be appealing to some, from a holistic standpoint it is superficial unless the inner voice is also trained. The intention behind this book is to assist those interested in finding, developing and using the Whole Voice.

Sound Thoughts

Another key to realizing our full vocal potential lies in understanding the "mind's voice," or the links between our spoken words, conscious intentions, and subconscious mind.

Sound is a magical force, and the voice is its vehicle. The words and sounds that we emit are generated by our mind's thoughts and intentions. The subconscious mind, which controls 90 percent of our body's functions and activities, actually responds to every thought, word, and sound we create. All vibrational energy follows thought. So when we give those thoughts and intentions vocalization, the energy created stimulates manifestation. For example, if we continually whine and complain that we can't do something, then what we manifest is not being able to do it, because our subconscious mind immediately responds to this negative vibration.

> *All vibrational energy follows thought.*

Through the sound of the voice, the subtle energy of thought-forms is intensified, grounded, and generated into the physical vibration, where it manifests. The more we voice something—positive or negative—in conjunction with that thought, the more quickly and powerfully that vibration will manifest within our lives. So if we choose to vocalize empowering words and sounds such as "I can do it" or "I quit smoking" or "I will no longer abuse my body," the subconscious mind responds to support and manifest these outcomes.

Fueled by the appropriate thoughts, our words and sounds can become extraordinary tools for manifestation and transformation, empowering the human voice as a healing instrument.

Vocal Responsibility

There is also the idea of personal responsibility when it comes to opening and using the voice—first, responsibility to ourselves, and then with regard to others. The voice is an expression of our character, our very soul, and everything we are. Therefore, it has great power to influence our lives and the lives of others. We can love, nurture, and support others with thoughtful and compassionate words and tones, helping them to find peace. We can also use our voice to wound others with thoughtless, insensitive, or abusive words, causing them to feel hurt, sad, afraid, or depressed.

Addressing this principle, *Sacred Sounds* author Ted Andrews states, "Control, discipline and awareness of speech is important. We must be cautious of casual or thoughtless remarks. The stronger and more developed we become, the greater the responsibility."

If we support ourselves with a positive attitude, self-love, and respect, we automatically create a foundation for peace and wellness to manifest. This is necessary to truly love, support, and respect others.

For example, we can get stressed, angry, and upset at times. Our voices then tend to gradually speed up and increase in volume. This is a natural phenomenon, and some would say it's healthy to "let off steam" in this manner. However, when we disrespect ourselves—and Omnipresent Spirit—by cursing, using profanity, and uttering crude, thoughtless, and irresponsible expressions, we only savage and negate ourselves. And when we direct these violent, verbal outbursts at another, we add even more unharmonious vibrations to the manic mix. Have you ever noticed how difficult it is to be present, loving, and able to focus your attention when you're upset?

More to the point, though, is our conscious awareness—and the intention that follows it—to "choose" words and expressions that truly serve us. It may seem like a minor transgression just to say "f*ck it" when we need an emotional release from some frustration but, in the big picture, does it really serve our highest good? Isn't there an equally effective expression of release? Some would surely argue no, claiming that the "F word" represents the ultimate release. But is this so, or just an excuse for trying to feel "strong" or look "tough?" Let's be honest. Is it a result of societal conditioning? Can we rise above our conditioning, influences, and peer pressures? Is it too difficult to discipline our vocal outbursts? Do we even want to? And why should we?

Certain words such as the "F word" and others are hot-wired into our subconscious minds and corrupt their original meanings. We can easily and unconsciously become entrapped by their deleterious effect on our hearts and minds. The "F word," for instance, tarnishes and demeans the beautiful act of lovemaking. It casually negates the natural, physical expression of love, and programs our subconscious mind—making us confused and in conflict about love and sex. Is this truly what we want?

Ultimately, we are solely responsible for our own thoughts, feelings, and vocalizations. However, if we take the time to practice mental discipline—by substituting positive and productive thoughts for negative and destructive ones—it becomes easier and healthier to vocalize our feelings appropriately. Not by repressing them, but by resonating with our feelings and expressing them in a controlled, clear, honest, and mature manner. Words that are spoken precisely and with real meaning produce greater benefits. This simple effort will result in manifesting more articulate, unifying, and effective expression and communication.

Consciousness of Expression Is an Expression of Consciousness

We don't have to pollute our consciousness with unhealthy thoughts, words, and sounds, if we have a clear intention not to do so. Although it might not be an *immediately* easy task to catch and re-direct every reactive feeling and expression, I've found it is well worth the effort.

I can recall when I first became aware of the potentially damaging effects that some of my vocal expressions could have on me and my loved ones. Some years ago, after a particularly difficult and stressful day at work, I got into an argument with my wife. In no time, I was ranting and raving, using profanity that I seldom use. I noticed my daughter, who was about 5 years old at the time, watching me with tears in her big, brown eyes. I stopped dead in my tracks, feeling that I had hurt her deeply. Although I hadn't directed my rage at her, I wondered what type of effect my angry expressions might have on her gentle spirit. I felt awful.

I set my intention to re-tune this frequency within myself and correct it. For me, eliminating crude talk and profanity from my vocabulary wasn't difficult because, thankfully, I've seldom used those types of expressions. More daunting for me was controlling my reactivity and vocal volume. Although it was—and sometimes still is—a struggle for me to be less reactive and more present in my heart when angry, the benefits to my health and relationships became immediately apparent. And though I've usually been prone to raising my voice when I am upset—having been affected by a "loud" family influence when growing up—in the last few years I seem to have made a lot of progress in keeping my inner peace (at least, according to my wife!).

Emotional Control Exercise

Here's an exercise I've used for some time that has helped greatly in giving me a "vibrationality check" and assisted me in achieving much improved emotional and vocal control: When you find yourself in an upsetting situation—feeling your patience dwindling and anger rising—first try to catch yourself before your feelings escalate and you say something that you might regret. Then imagine that you're in the presence of someone you really love, admire, and respect. (This person may be from the past or present.) Ask yourself how you would feel using that volume or tone of voice, or saying that word. How would you appear to him or her? How would he or she feel? And what would he or she think?

This perspective acts as a kinder reminder and reality check for self-appraisal of your expressiveness. Are you honoring yourself (and anyone else present)? Are you truly expressing your highest truth for your highest good? How do you feel? Are you mastering "emotionally mature mouth control"?

If you still feel a need for emotional release, I would suggest toning a loud vowel sound (if in an appropriate environment). Another good release is to exclaim some nonsensical word such as "Flerbit!" or "Shreeet!" This process will effect a satisfactory release while shifting you into a humorous or lighter mood. Use whatever works and have fun.

≈

The Catch

Another way in which we subtly sabotage ourselves is with common catch phrases. Although most may be harmless, there are some that feed back a harsh or negative message to our subconscious mind—for example, "I can kill two birds with one stone." An alternative phrase might be, "I can feed two birds with one seed." Another cliché says, "There is more than one way to skin a cat." I'm sure conscious cat-lovers would prefer saying, "There is more than one way to trim a cat," "train a cat," or "love a cat." You get the idea. Can you think of some common phrases that would benefit from some "rewarding re-wording"? Developing more conscious awareness of the words we use and how we speak them is essential to maximize the potentials inherent within the voice, and ultimately, for accessing our Whole Voice. The reward for practicing mental and emotional discipline through vocal control is freedom of spirit. Understanding how our vocal expressions affect our body, mind, and soul—as well as how they impact others—is a most vital lesson. From it we can learn how to restore homeostasis to the mind-body and use the human voice as the ultimate healing instrument.

> *The reward for practicing mental and emotional discipline through vocal control is freedom of spirit.*

(((((7)))))

Vocalization Preparation

If you don't touch the rope, you won't ring the bell.

—English proverb

Before we can make fullest use of the wonderful instrument that is the human voice, we need to first take a few minutes to prepare it. We need to warm up the voice and create a solid foundation from which to maximize its expression. Similar to the way body stretching helps us to obtain the most flexibility before exercising, likewise we need to prepare and stretch the vocal cords and related systems before fully expressing the voice. The first important step in this process and one of the fundamentals of good vocal production is breathing—specifically, diaphragmatic breathing.

Diaphragmatic Breathing

To maximize the prana—or life force energy of the breath—it is vital to practice this simple breathing technique. Any good singing teacher, diction coach, or voice coach worth his/her salt will always teach diaphragmatic breathing for optimal vocal prowess. It's not only essential for the best voice production, but may indeed add a few years to our lives by improving oxygenation in the bloodstream. Thus, I recommend that it be learned and practiced daily until it becomes habit.

Diaphragmatic Breathing Exercises

There are two simple exercises for easily learning diaphragmatic breathing:

1. Lie down on the floor; place one hand on your stomach and feel your stomach rise and fall—quite naturally—as you breathe from your diaphragm. Then sit up straight and continue breathing slowly from your stomach. When we sleep, the body naturally breathes this way to conserve energy. This is how we should always breathe.

2. While standing, sitting, or lying down, place one hand, palm toward you, on your lower abdomen. Without lifting your chest or shoulders, inhale deeply, while pushing your hand and lower abdomen outwards simultaneously. Then, while exhaling, pull your hand and lower abdomen inwards, keeping your hand pressed firmly on your abdomen. Repeat this process until it feels comfortable and rhythmic. Inhale—hand and tummy out; exhale—hand and tummy in; keep repeating. (Be careful not to lift your chest or shoulders while inhaling; this may result in shallow breathing, the incorrect way most of us breathe unconsciously and unhealthfully.)

≈

Although it usually comes easily for most people, if diaphragmatic breathing doesn't immediately feel natural to you, be patient and persistent. It is crucial for sound health, and in time this method will begin to feel comfortable, for this is the way we once breathed naturally as babies. Most of us unlearned this natural form of breathing sometime during childhood after being subjected to threats, shame, punishment, and so forth—from parents, siblings, teachers, and the like. Feelings generated by these types of actions and behavior have caused us to breathe shallowly, and are connected to fight-or-flight responses that do not support our health and well-being. So there are many supportive health benefits associated with learning and maintaining diaphragmatic breathing.

Good Habits

Some factors that can dramatically affect the sound of your voice and detract from its optimal capabilities are attitude, breath, movement, thoughts and emotions, tension and stress, diet, volume, overuse, and improper usage. To avoid the pitfalls and handicaps associated with these factors and maximize the potentials of your voice, I suggest the following:

≈ Instill in yourself an open and positive attitude, along with a committed intention to learn how to best use your vocal instrument.

≈ Until it becomes second nature, monitor your breath to make sure you are breathing deeply and diaphragmatically before exercising the voice.

≈ Do some vocal warm-up exercises every day—preferably in the morning—so that you may prepare the voice for active use without straining. (While showering or driving is often convenient.)

≈ Do not strain the voice by overuse, or using too much volume: yelling, shouting, screaming, over-singing, singing, or toning outside of your normal vocal range, talking too loud or too much.

≈ Get enough rest and sleep to rejuvenate both the body and the voice.

≈ Meditate. Develop spiritual awareness.

≈ Combine vocal sounding with physical body movement and exercising. (This may include humming, grunting, sighing, using vowels sounds, or any releasing types of vocal sounds; see Chapter 8.)

≈ Establish a disciplined and regular routine for vocal practices.

≈ Avoid overeating and any unhealthy foods that contribute to sluggishness, fatigue, and lack of energy, and those that create excessive mucous (sugar, alcohol, meat, dairy products, and processed foods).

Habits work more constantly and with greater force than reasoning.

—John Locke

Good habits—along with conscious breathing and regular vocal practices—will go a long way in supporting and strengthening the voice.

The Toning Vowels

One of the very best vocal practices involves using the vowels, specifically what I call the *toning vowels*. The sounds that resonate the voice most effectively are vowel sounds. Whether we are speaking, singing, or toning, the vowels facilitate the fullest opening of the voice by allowing the maximum flow of breath to support vocal sounding. *Sounding* is another word for *toning,* and the toning vowels give us a clear, strong foundation for developing the voice.

In the English language, the vowels are: A, E, I, O, and U. In terms of letters, they make up the heart of the alphabet. How many words can you make with no vowels in them? This resonant family of five empowers the alphabet, the extraordinary communication tool that creates language, literature, art, and so forth. Similarly, vowels are the heart of sound and toning.

Before we can make the best use of the toning vowels, however, we need to simplify them by removing the diphthongs. A diphthong is a combination vowel, or two connected vowels pronounced as one. For example, there are two diphthongs in our five vowels: I and U. When we slow down our pronunciation of the I vowel, we hear the sound as "AH-EE"—two vowel sounds. Likewise, when we slow down the U vowel, we hear "EE-OO." To simplify the pronunciations and better focus the sound energy, we can tone "AH" and "OO," instead of I and U, for these two vowel sounds. Thus the pure sounds of our five vowels are: "AY–EE–AH–OH–OO."

By the way, if your primary language is one other than English or you grew up in another English-speaking country, you may have learned the vowels differently from the way they are taught in the United States. There may be no diphthongs present, nor may the vowels be pronounced in quite the same way—and their order may be different, as well. No matter. Just tone the pure vowels in any manner and order that feels comfortable to you while adhering to the same sound principles.

To complete our full set of toning vowels we need to add a sixth vowel sound to the group: "UH." This additional vowel contributes grounding and added resonance to the voice. It rhymes with "run" or "fun," and should not be confused with the "AH" vowel sound (amen or mirage). We now have the toning vowels: AY–EE–AH–OH–OO–UH.

The Siren Vowel Exercise

A very useful vocal warm-up exercise that is one of the easiest and most effective for opening up the voice is the Siren Vowel Exercise. I call it so because, while doing it, the voice sounds somewhat similar to a siren. Any adept voice coach or singing teacher will use some variation of this exercise in teaching students techniques for optimal vocal preparation. I've used it in various forms since I was 18 years old and first studying voice. The Siren Vowel Exercise is great for strengthening and developing the voice in any context (speaking, singing, chanting, or toning).

Begin by finding the lowest pitch or note that you can tone comfortably without straining. While breathing diaphragmatically, sound the first toning vowel—"AY"—at that vocal pitch. In one breath, gradually move up in pitch, from low to high, as you continue toning this first vowel sound. When you reach the top of your vocal range, or highest pitch, come back down without pausing to your lowest pitch, where you began. You will slowly be releasing your breath as you tone the vowel sound from low to high to low. Repeat this same process with each toning vowel. Be sure to complete each vowel in one breath.

If you run out of breath before returning to your lowest note, there is one of two reasons for this, and both can be easily remedied. The first possibility is that you didn't start with a deep diaphragmatic breath to support your voice adequately. The second is that you may have simply gone too slowly through the steps of the vowel toning. Whichever the case, begin again, being sure to start with a good breath, and then move through the exercise rapidly enough—but not too quickly—to complete the process properly. After you've practiced the Siren Vowel Exercise a few times, it will become readily apparent how to easily execute and flow with it.

In terms of the time necessary to adequately prepare the voice with this exercise, I would recommend at least five minutes. You may run through all the toning vowels consecutively for five minutes, or you may spend one minute with each vowel—one at a time—if you choose. Have fun with it. Making it a regular part of your morning routine will clear and strengthen your voice, energize you, and create a strong vibrational foundation for the day. During your morning shower and while driving your car are usually convenient times for this vocal practice, and will be well worth the time and effort you put in.

≈

Hands-On Sound Exercise

Developing a deeper connectedness and intimacy with your voice will greatly enhance your vocal prowess, vibrational awareness, and overall resonance. One of the ways in which you can easily begin establishing this connection is by using your hands while doing toning exercises. In addition to their inherent ability to project healing vibrations, the hands can also be used as resonators to receive and feel sound vibrations. An excellent way to experience this is by placing your hands on various areas of the body while toning different sounds.

For example, as you tone a vowel sound during the Siren Vowel Exercise, place the palm of one hand on your lower abdomen and the other on your solar plexus or upper abdomen. Notice the vibrations of the sound against your hands. Which hand feels a stronger vibration? Is it easier to feel during your lower toning sounds, or the higher ones? Imagine that your hands are microphones, and notice what you feel.

Now, leaving one hand on your solar plexus, move the lower hand up to the heart or chest area. Pressing gently against your breastbone or sternum, tone another vowel and notice how the sound vibrations feel against your hands. Does it feel the same as the last vowel sound? Is this vowel any easier to tone or feel? Or more difficult? Which hand feels a stronger vibration this time?

Continue toning the remaining vowels in the Siren Vowel Exercise while changing your hand placement positions: one hand on the chest, the other on the neck or throat area; one hand on the throat, the other on the crown of the head; one hand on the head, the other on the solar plexus; one hand on the chest, the other on the face or cheeks. What do you notice? Are any vowels easier or more comfortable to tone than others? Did any resistance come up for you during any of the vowels? Were you aware of any energy shifts in your body while toning? Did the sound energy move up or down your body with the pitch of your voice? How does your voice feel now?

> *In proportion to your intention and commitment to resonance, you'll become "tuned in" to your signature frequency.*

As you practice this exercise regularly, your awareness of the connection between your voice and your body will become expanded and enhanced. Energy blocks and areas of resistance will gradually release with your sounding, and you will find a greater facility, range, timbre, and strength in your voice. In proportion to your intention and commitment to resonance, you'll become more "tuned in" to your signature frequency and the sound of your soul.

≈

Resonant Breathing

In addition to diaphragmatic breathing, another important preparatory foundation for toning is the use of the breath to balance and ground the body-mind. Resonant Breathing is an integrative process that concentrates and amplifies our energy, focus of attention, and vocal capacity. Through this conscious breathing technique we can more easily create a vibrational resonance that moves us toward transformation and healing, both inner and outer.

When we are lacking the proper resonance in our bodies, minds, and souls, we are out of touch with the "soul-self." We experience feelings of fear, confusion, and separation from our Source. This dissonance and lack of body-mind harmony leads to illness and disease, which reminds us to return to resonance and oneness. Upon experiencing balance and alignment with our soul-self, or true self, we no longer feel fear and separation. We can return home in resonance with our Source. This is our ultimate healing and liberation.

Resonant Breathing initiates the integrative healing process, for it can balance the left- and right-brain hemispheres to create a sense of unity within ourselves. Other body-mind polarities often in need of balance and integration include the active and the passive, the sympathetic and the parasympathetic, the masculine and the feminine, the yin and the yang, and the inspirational breath of life and the expirational breath of death. All of these polarities can be brought into balance with the rhythmic pattern of the Resonant Breathing Exercise, which coheres a balanced state of consciousness that profoundly enhances the vibrational healing process.

> *Lack of mind-body harmony leads to illness and disease, which reminds us to return to resonance and oneness.*

The Resonant Breathing Exercise

This powerful technique is made up of three components. The first two are for balancing the left- and right-brain hemispheres and integrating the body-mind polarities. The third component is for stabilizing and grounding your signature frequency: preparing the vibrational energy field for transformation. Once learned and practiced, the whole exercise can be completed in a total of 21 breaths (seven breaths per component) and within 90 to 120 seconds.

Component 1

- ≈ Assume a comfortable and relaxed position, with your eyes closed.

- ≈ Gently breathe, diaphragmatically, through the nose.

- ≈ Focus your attention at the tip of your left foot; inhale while imagining the breath coming in through your foot, up the left leg and left side of your body, in through your left nostril, and up to the center of your forehead.

- ≈ Hold your breath for a second at the forehead; release it— following the same path down the body with your exhalation— out through the left nostril, down the left side of the body, down the left leg, and out through the tip of your left foot.

≈ Repeat this part of the process two more times, for a total of three "left-side" breaths.

≈ Shift your attention to your right side and follow the same method as the left—imagining your breath drawing in through the tip of your right foot while inhaling, and coming up the right side of the body, in through the right nostril, and up to the center of the forehead.

≈ Hold your breath for a second at the forehead, and then release it in the same manner, down the right side of the body and out through the tip of the right foot.

≈ Again, repeat this two more times for a total of three "right-side" breaths—or a combined total of six breaths.

≈ For the seventh and final breath of this component, imagine the breath coming in through both feet, coming up both legs, up the center of the body, in through both nostrils and up to the center of the forehead.

≈ Hold it for a second, then release the breath—as if from your forehead—through both nostrils simultaneously, with a short expulsion of breath and a sigh-like sound. This completes the first component.

Note: Although you may do so if you choose, it is not necessary to hold the opposite nostril closed with your finger—yoga style—while breathing through either nostril. A clear intention is sufficient.

Component 2

≈ As in the last component, imagine your breath coming in through the tip of your right foot, up the right side, in through the right nostril and up to the center of the forehead.

≈ This time, however, after holding it for a second, release your exhalation through the left nostril, continuing down the left side of the body, and out through the left foot.

≈ Drawing in your second breath, come up the left side of the body, in through the left nostril and up to the center of the forehead. After holding it for a second, exhale through the right nostril, continuing down the right side of the body and out through the right foot.

≈ This cross-breathing technique should continue for a total of six breaths (three in each direction).

≈ The seventh and final breath in this component is again done in the same way as the first component: Inhale through the tips of both feet. Imagine the energy of the breath coming up the center of the body, in through both nostrils to the center of the forehead; hold for a second, then release your exhalation through the nose with a short expulsion of breath and a sigh-like sound.

This completes the second component.

The first two components of the Resonant Breathing Exercise, when done properly, will take only 30 to 40 seconds each.

Component 3

≈ As in the seventh breath of the first two components, imagine inhaling through your feet, drawing in the breath up the center of the body, in through both nostrils to the center of the forehead.

≈ After holding it for a second, release your breath—as if from the sixth chakra in the center of the forehead—out through the mouth, gently and simultaneously sighing the first toning-vowel-sound: "AY." (If you are unfamiliar with the chakras, further information is given in Chapter 10.)

≈ Inhale your second breath in the same manner as the first, except upon reaching the exhalation point at the forehead, shift to sighing the second toning-vowel-sound: "EE."

≈ Continue the same process with each of the remaining toning-vowel-sounds: "AH," "OH," "OO," "UH." One vowel for each out-breath.

≈ After completing the sixth breath using the "UH" vowel, continue with the seventh breath in the same way as the sixth, repeating the "UH" vowel. However, upon reaching the exhalation point at the forehead, sigh into the "UH" vowel from the high end, or "top," of your voice and "ride" your pitch down—lower and lower, until reaching the lowest note you can comfortably tone.

≈ While toning this last vowel, simultaneously imagine the sound and breath flowing out from the sixth chakra at the center of the forehead, and moving down the whole body through all the chakras, down to the base of the spine. This will assist you in fully grounding yourself at the first chakra.

≈ Upon reaching this root energy center, fully release all the oxygen from your lungs. Open your eyes (unless proceeding into a meditation or toning process), take a deep diaphragmatic breath, and continue breathing normally.

This completes the Resonant Breathing Exercise in a total of 21 breaths, which should take less than two minutes. Notice enhanced body-mind alignment and resonance, as your brain hemispheres and body polarities will now be in balance.

The conscious breathing exercise outlined here is highly recommended before any vocal, toning, or healing practice, as it focuses attention, integrates vibrational energy, prepares the voice, opens the sixth chakra for enhanced intuition, and clears the way for body-mind transformation.

≈

The time and energy spent on warming up the voice and preparing the body-mind for transformation is well worth the effort. Just as we take care in preparing our automobile for a trip by filling it up with gas, and checking the oil, brakes, tires, and air pressure, don't our voices and bodies deserve the same care? Not to mention our minds and souls.

The easily executed practices of Diaphragmatic Breathing, Good Habits, and the Siren Vowel and Resonant Breathing Exercises will establish a strong foundation for any type of vocalizing or sound healing work. You will obtain unlimited mileage from their use.

(((((8)))))

The Three Toning Sounds

A sigh is a silent shout.

—Wayne Perry

Back in the days when I was first fascinated with reading philosophy and mysticism, I read some words of wisdom that have stayed with me. I don't recall who said them, but I'll attempt to paraphrase: *The simple truths are the most valuable and profound. If you have to weed through complicated layers of information, philosophies, and a lot of intellectual mumbo-jumbo to get at the truth, it's probably a load of crap.* Though somewhat blunt, this has proved to be very true and helpful for me to remember in studying life's mysteries. It seems to be a tendency of the mind to often overanalyze and complicate useful information. The knowledge that has proven to be the most profound and useful to me in my search for truth has usually revealed itself through the beauty of simplicity.

Simple Essence

Simplicity is fundamental to toning. Although we can certainly enhance and perfect various techniques to further develop a mastery of toning skills, as with any endeavor, its very essence is simplicity. For instance, we can observe the natural use of our voices on any given day and notice the simple, yet vital, sounds that we often release: moaning, groaning, sighing, murmuring, whimpering, giggling, laughing, crying, shouting, screaming, snickering, sniffling, sneezing, coughing, burping, humming, yawning, grunting.

We may not refer to it as such, but this is all toning. If we recall our toning definition from earlier, we can see that these examples of "spontaneous sounding," whether done consciously or unconsciously, fall under the category of toning. When we add a conscious intention to our toning, we simply energize and enhance the natural vibrational healing potential inherent in the sounds of the voice for optimal results.

The Three Rs

To assist us in making the best use of our toning sounds, it may be helpful to explore their basic components. I have found that there are three fundamental sounds. For easy understanding, I categorize them as the Three Rs:

1. Relaxing sounds.
2. Releasing sounds.
3. Regenerative sounds.

Let's define and explore each of these three sounds in which we can find full therapeutic expression through the natural power of vocal toning.

1. Relaxing Sounds

The purpose of sounds that relax is to calm and soothe the body. The process of vocally producing relaxing sounds is to utter quiet and soft tones within the overall volume of the sounding. For example, if we wanted to lull a baby to sleep with the voice, we would hum or tone soft, gentle vowels, or sounds that would support the baby in relaxation and sleep. In this instance, a lullaby is obviously more appropriate than a loud rock song! Relaxation sounds are generally the easiest of the three toning sounds.

Relaxing Sounds Exercise

Here is a toning exercise that you can do to relax the body. Sit upright; breathe deeply with your eyes closed while imagining oxygen flowing freely to every part of the body that needs relaxation. After a few deep breaths, allow your voice to make soft, sustained "aahs," "oohs," or humming to assist in deeper relaxation. After a few more breaths, notice which parts of the body (limbs, muscles, joints) need the most relaxing, and consciously tone these soft sounds directly into those specific areas. Allow those body parts to be calmed, be soothed, and feel more relaxed with each successive breath and tone. Continue as long as necessary to fully relax your body.

≈

2. Releasing Sounds

The purpose of releasing sounds is to clear and cleanse the body. The process of vocally producing releasing sounds is to use enough volume and breath to increase the flow and release of vibrational energy. This is further enhanced with the primary use of vowels. For example, if a large person were to step on your foot with all of his/her weight, how would you express or release the pain and discomfort? Most likely, you wouldn't exclaim, "Bam!" or "Beep!" These are not appropriate release sounds (at least on planet Earth!). More likely you would express, "Ow!" "Ooh!" or something of that nature.

This example shows us that some vocal sounds are more appropriate than others in different circumstances, but all release sounds seem to have three things in common: vowels, volume, and breath. Specifically, a vocal emphasis on one or more vowel sounds facilitates a better integration of increased volume and life force energy (breath) for optimal releasing. Whether you are releasing physical, emotional, or mental stress and pain, the sound principles are the same.

With regard to volume, don't stress or strain your voice. This is not "primal scream therapy." If you repeatedly use too much volume, you may damage your voice and vocal cords. Use just enough volume to feel a shift in your energy. Louder than speaking, but not quite shouting, is usually sufficient for adequate release. Allow your feelings and intuition to guide you.

If you are releasing a deep or painful longstanding issue, it might require a bit more volume. If it's a temporary or minor issue, use less volume. **Note:** Toning release work is essentially the only type of toning in which extra volume is needed. Most all other toning does not require much volume and too much may even be counterproductive.

Releasing Sounds Exercise #1

To affect the release of pain or discomfort with this method, tone through all the releasing sounds mentioned at the beginning of the chapter (moaning, sighing, and so on) one at a time, while noticing the difference in how each sound feels physically and emotionally. Then select the sounds and feelings that you would most like to release at this time. This works best if you sit with your eyes closed and imagine yourself feeling the feelings associated with each releasing sound as you emphasize your vowels, volume, and breath, while releasing the sound.

For instance, you may imagine feeling the tension that might be held in particular muscles of the body after physically working out at the gym, or being emotionally stressed at your job. As you breathe deeply into the tightness within these muscles, release a deep sigh—emphasizing the "AAH" sound—to facilitate the release of the tension from the muscles. Repeat this a few times, as needed, and then move to another feeling and type of release sound.

≈

Imagine what the state of your body might be if you never expressed any releasing sounds when feeling pain! We often repress our natural and instinctive sounds of release because of social pressures, parental upbringing, and other influences that contribute to our personal inhibitions and associated disempowerment. Men, in particular, have added difficulties because of social customs that dictate that it's more desirable to be the "strong, silent type," and that men shouldn't express too many feelings— let alone sounds!

Women generally are more expressive and less inhibited, and perhaps this is—at least in part—why they live longer than men. I have noticed in years of leading toning workshops and seminars—both nationally and internationally—that the women usually outnumber the men. However, we needn't be restricted by gender roles, parental and societal influences, or anything else on our toning journey and in the use of releasing sounds.

Releasing Sounds Exercise #2

Another good toning exercise for releasing pent-up tension and stress is as follows: Stand straight, with feet shoulder-width apart (approximately 18 inches). Keeping the body loose and intuitively moving with the sound, release each vowel sound (pure vowels, without diphthongs) over and over again in short bursts of breath and raised volume. Example: "AY–EE–AH–OH–OO! AY–EE–AH–OH–OO!" Do 15 to 20 repetitions. Stop, close your eyes, and feel the energy moving through your body for 20 to 30 seconds while breathing deeply. Notice any changes in the way you feel from before you began the exercise. Observe if you feel more grounded, focused, clear. Begin again, this time adding a consonant in front of the each vowel: "HAY–HEE–HAH–HOH–HOO," or "SHAY–SHEE–SHAH–SHOH–SHOO," and repeat the same process. Do five or six complete sets of vowel repetitions, substituting a different consonant in front of each vowel sound for each set. Don't forget to pause, breathe, and feel between each set. Continue this process until you feel a satisfactory release from the tension and stress.

≈

Although toning release work is most effective when done standing— and in a space that may accommodate any movements that might better facilitate releasing—this is also a great exercise for de-stressing the body while in your car and stuck in traffic. Just roll up the windows and wail! This type of toning is a great way to clear any confused or blocked emotions when feeling overwhelmed by them. (For more detailed information on deeper emotional release work, see Chapter 18.)

In terms of the time necessary for successfully completing a toning release session, it may depend on several factors: how often you do the exercise, how much energy you put into it, how deep the issues are that you are working with, and how many issues there are. If you are the type of person who gets really involved and you throw yourself completely into a process, you may do the exercise in longer sessions, but maybe less frequently (say, once or twice a week). On the other hand, if you are just working on releasing simple, everyday stresses and tensions, or haven't an abundance of time on any given day, you may choose to spend just a few minutes daily building up your release practice. Do what works best for your situation and lifestyle.

3. Regenerative Sounds.

The purpose of regenerative sounds is to strengthen, rebuild and heal the mind-body. Whereas relaxation and releasing sounds create an environment for healing and assist the therapeutic process, regenerative sounds are the truly healing sounds. These frequencies are

> *You can learn to encode your intent into the particular sound you are toning.*

perhaps the most mysterious and misunderstood of all the toning sounds. They include a wide array of powerful vocal sounding principles and techniques that may be grouped into five basic categories for better understanding:

1. Harmonic sounds pertain to the use of vocal harmonics and overtones (as regenerative frequencies). Of the five types of regenerative frequencies, the practice of vocal overtoning may be the most vibrationally effective sounding technique. When combined with any or all of the other four types of sounds, the healing power of regeneration may be further enhanced. Because the methodology associated with overtoning as a healing modality is so comprehensive and important, I have devoted an entire chapter (Chapter 12) to the techniques and exercises involved.

2. Tuned sounds are those that are pitched or tuned for the support of specific body systems. They work with balancing the individual needs of one's personal vibrations and signature frequency. A musical instrument, tuning fork, pitch pipe, or other tuning device may be used in assisting the voice in toning the appropriate pitch or frequency. When the body-mind is brought into vibrational balance and resonance with tuned vocal sounds, the body can actually heal itself.

3. Coherent sounds are based on the principle that sound can communicate a variety of thoughts and emotions. Certain types of sounds tend to create a sense of order or coherency. They stimulate feelings of safety, trust, gratitude, love, and joy. This may be opposed to chaotic sounds, which tend to create feelings of paranoia, distrust, fear, anger, and hatred. By making vocal sounds associated with uplifting and coherent feelings, we can help to create a psychological order and sense of wellness within ourselves and others.

4. Encoded sounds are those infused with a specific intention and consciousness. Because sound is a carrier wave for intention, you can learn to encode your intent into the particular sound you are toning. The more you focus your intention—with concentration—into your toning sound, the more effective the encoding will be. As we grow in our understanding of sound healing principles, the use and importance of encoding sound becomes more apparent.

5. Sacred sounds are generally prayers, chants, and mantras, and are mostly used in association with various ancient, cultural, and/or spiritual practices. Usually containing tones or words of power, sacred sounds rely on the faith and belief of the one speaking, chanting, or toning the mystically empowered frequencies. However, any sound may be sacred based upon the intention and consciousness behind it.

Any or all of these regenerative sounds may be used separately or in combinations to facilitate sound healing and personal transformation. They may be directed into any areas of the body that need resonance and support. Results can be attained through patient practice and are enhanced by the clarity of your intention, the state of your consciousness, and the facility with which your sounds are employed and directed.

> *Any sound may be sacred based upon the intention and consciousness behind it.*

The application of regenerative sounds is best incorporated after doing the aforementioned release sounding, serving to fill any void left by the releasing process. This will then enable rebuilding and regeneration to take place in those body-mind areas and assist in achieving and maintaining sound health.

Recorded Sounds

Regenerative sounds may be recorded and listened to regularly for ongoing vibrational support. However, the very process of recording, as well as listening to any sounds—whether digital or analog—automatically "freezes," isolates, and affects the vibrational and harmonic content within the sounds. Although not as fully beneficial as toning or listening to live vocal sounds, recordings of the sounds can still be an effective and convenient method for sound healing. But how do we find recordings of regenerative sounds? Which ones are best?

Sound healing has already entered the awareness of recording artists who are, in many cases, untrained in this field of study and its healing application. So whenever possible, try to listen to a recording before you purchase it (nowadays, most stores have listening stations to accommodate customers) or consult with a sound therapist for recommendations. If you still are unsure of the uses and benefits of a recording, you may use the Three Rs for guidance.

Sound Advice

Here are some tips to serve you in finding the most appropriate sounds to listen to:

≈ If you are simply looking for sounds or music that you can relax to, select anything that assists you in feeling calmed and soothed. If you don't feel peaceful and relaxed while listening to a recording, don't buy it, even if the liner notes claim that some scientific technology is being used for inducing relaxation. Trust yourself.

≈ If you're looking for sounds to assist you in the release process, listen for sounds, chants, or music that help you to feel energized and uplifted. If the sounds or rhythms inspire you to hum, sing, tone, move, or dance, it's probably a good bet they can support any needed releasing.

≈ Finding good recordings of regenerative sounds may be a bit more difficult. In our culture, most of us tend to be "lazy listeners." We're preprogrammed since childhood—mostly through exposure to radio and television—to be used to and comfortable with sounds and music that may be vibrationally unhealthy, and we may not have the necessary time, information, or interest level to make an informed choice.

I usually recommend following one's intuition in making these types of choices. But although I support trusting one's feelings, there is an important issue that needs to be considered: We may sometimes be drawn to sounds that are not healthy or good for us. These sounds may feel appealing, intriguing, beautiful, or even feel subconsciously "safe" to us, but could be deleterious to our resonance and wellness. This is similar to the way some of us are attracted to people, foods, or substances that don't support our optimal well-being. On the other hand, we may reject or resist sounds that could offer the most benefit to us.

> *We may sometimes be drawn to sounds that are not healthy or good for us.*

My suggestion in dealing with this dilemma is to take the time to listen to a variety of potentially regenerative sounds, and do a little research to find out which ones may support your personal needs and unique signature frequency. This may be accomplished through a diagnostic voice analysis with a qualified sound therapist, or through subtle-energy alternatives such as dowsing, muscle-testing, or intuitive development. (These options will be discussed in more detail in Chapter 13 and Chapter 14.) Ultimately, we need to accept the relativity of our perceptions to sound in the context of healing. Our environment, attitude, and receptivity, as well as our expectations and beliefs, have much to do with the outcome.

Sound can be uniquely personal in its effects, and what might be healing for one person might offer nothing to another. Your responses to sound are an interaction between the sound, the sound maker, and the vast complexities of your own signature vibration.

However you choose to use the Three Rs—for your own wellness and transformation, in the service of others, or for guidance in listening support—be gentle and patient with yourself. Have fun toning them. Often, just being present, receptive, and resonant can open new dimensions of sonic awareness. In upcoming chapters, we will explore in more detail additional toning exercises and sound healing principles for listening to your inner tones and voicing your soul.

(((((9)))))

Name Toning: What's in a Name?

There is a great secret hidden in a name,
be it the name of a person or thing,
and it is formed in relation to the past,
present and future conditions of its object….
All mystery is hidden in name.

—Hazrat Inayat Khan

The Mysticism of Sound

The specific sound that identifies each one of us, and distinguishes us from one another, is commonly referred to as our name. Great vibrational power lies within our name. But are we aware of it? Can we feel it? How are we affected by it? What is its secret and significance? These questions may be answered by taking a new perspective on how we view our name.

The name that identifies us—particularly, our given name, or first name—has a vibrational effect on us because we hear it repeatedly. We usually hear it more than we say it, so we are constantly receiving this vibration. Hearing our name spoken or called by others has a powerful effect because vocal sound is a carrier wave for consciousness. This repetition of our name is one of several ways in which the name has a vibrational influence. Another is the way in which we receive the sound of our name.

Do you like your name? Does hearing your name trigger certain feelings and emotions? How are you influenced and affected by the feelings and the intentions of a person saying or calling your name? When you hear your name spoken by strangers, do you feel the same way as when hearing it from family members? Are we affected by the consciousness of our parents or those who named us? And if so, how?

The practice of "name toning" may lead you to some surprising answers to these questions. It may also assist you in healing any vibrational toxicity held within your name and mind-body.

Vibrational Toxicity

As our basic essence is vibrational in nature, it is inevitable that the sound of our names has some sort of impact on us. Because conscious intention is encoded within every word and sound that is uttered, the extent to which we are affected by the sound resonated to us through our name is in proportion to our receptivity and openness. Because we are the most open and receptive during our early childhood, during this time of life is usually when we are particularly vulnerable to emotional and vibrational toxicity. This toxicity inhibits the body's overall resonance and may create dissonance within your signature frequency.

> *As our basic essence is vibrational in nature, it is inevitable that the sound of our names has some sort of impact on us.*

Because we have such a strong personal identification with it, our first name may store these unhealthy energies. Many are unaware of these vibrational influences and unconsciously carry them in their minds and bodies for their entire lives. Others are sensitive to them and may change their names to free themselves from the uncomfortable energies they experience. Although this may be helpful, it may not be necessary, if we can redefine our names, and reprogram our attitudes and reactions to them.

Childhood Influences

We may all recall incidents in our childhood when we were scolded by a parent or family member for something we did (or didn't!) do. Remember the ways that your name was expressed and emphasized: "Wayne, put that down!" "Wayne, what did you do?" "Wayne, sit still!" "Wayne, be quiet!" "Waaa-aaayne!!" Just fill in the blanks with your name: "_____, stop hitting your sister!" "_____, take your finger out of your nose!" "_____, if I have to come over there, you'll be sorry!" "_____, go to your room!" You get the idea. It's no wonder that we may want to change our name, or may have difficulty loving ourselves!

Our parents may have meant well in their caring and concern for our well-being, but may have been ill-equipped to always respond to our every action with the optimal patience, equanimity, nurturing support, and loving guidance that we may have needed at the time. The results of these often threatening, angry, judgmental expressions by our parents (or guardians, family members, teachers, and so forth) are an emotional and vibrational toxicity that becomes unconsciously infused into our name. Throughout our childhood, and frequently, into our adult years as well, we have absorbed the negative effects of this toxic residue, which may greatly affect our body-mind health and wellness.

Name Toning

So how can we overcome these old frequency patterns and negative influences? Changing our name is one option, but it may be just a bandage. Though a name change may shift a frequency and help us to feel better with ourselves, it doesn't change or release stored frequencies from the past. How do we redefine and reprogram our name without changing it? How can we facilitate the necessary frequency shifts to free ourselves from the bondage of past influences and vibrational toxicity? The answer to these questions is *name toning*.

The name toning exercise is a simple, fun, and effective healing practice that I've developed, used, and taught in my sound healing workshops for some years. The process is essentially a release exercise that uses, primarily, the first name—or any name holding an emotional charge—as a vehicle for releasing blocked or toxic energy from the body-mind.

The Name Toning Exercise

Begin by recalling any names, name derivatives, or nicknames you were called by family or friends. Unless you were routinely called by your last name, always refer to your first name when doing this process. Notice which names felt hurtful or uncomfortable. Notice the way they sounded or were pronounced and emphasized. Who spoke them? Recall who may have said your name in the most impactful or derogatory manner. Was it primarily friends or family? Was it your parents? One parent? An older brother or sister? All of the above? After you've recognized the most significant people and issues involved, close your eyes, sit comfortably, and prepare to go deeper.

Remember what thoughts and feelings came up for you when you heard your name called or spoken. Without repressing or negating your feelings, create the intention to sincerely learn from, and release the past and any pain associated with it. In most cases, our parents and others whom we feel hurt us were simply insensitive or unconscious of their actions and their effects on us. It's always the healthiest choice to forgive and bless them.

≈

Childhood Names

Recall any childhood names you were given that have an "emotional charge" in them. This includes any odd pronunciations of your name, derivatives, or nicknames. How many are there? Identify and sound them out, one at a time. For example, some derivatives of the name *William* are Will, Willy, Bill, and Billy. Derivatives of the name *Patricia* are Pat, Patty, Trish, and Trisha. A nickname could be almost anything: Spike, Bubba, Buddy, Shorty, Slim, Bony, Chubby, Squirt, Stinky, Pokey, Missy. Keep in mind that you're looking for names that you were routinely called, and that had a "negative charge" for you—not nicknames of endearment.

If you don't recall any nicknames or derivatives of your name, simply focus on your name as you heard and felt it, and proceed with the exercise as indicated. The principles and practices are the same.

The Charges

Once you've completed this identification portion of the exercise, with your eyes closed, begin sounding the negatively charged name. Don't rush through this. Whether you're toning one name or five, spend at least a couple of minutes on each name. Methodically tone each syllable of each name, emphasizing the vowels and volume in the same way that you recall hearing and feeling them when you were a child. Begin with the names that are the least comfortable to hear, sound, and feel. Tone through each name and sound, noticing which emotions come up for you and being careful not to resist feeling any of them.

As you allow yourself to patiently go through this process, you will gradually be able to resonate easily with the names, sounds, and feelings, and experience a natural release of the "charged" or blocked energy associated with the past. Let any feelings of childhood pain, grief, shame, or anger flow through your body and be released without resistance. Many people carry this resistance and "old pain" in their names and bodies all of their lives. This need no longer be necessary with the practice of the transformational Name Toning Exercise.

Childlike Faith in Childhood's End

"Should be seen
and not heard,"
A child in fear
can't feel assured.
Sound your truth
my little friend,
Have childlike faith
in childhood's end.
Through lives & times
we have roamed,
Now it's time
to journey home.
To heal our hearts
and spirits mend,
Takes childlike faith
in childhood's end...

—Wayne Perry

Healing Your Name

After you feel complete with the release portion of this process, it's time to move on to the final stage of name toning: healing your name. With your eyes still closed, slowly sound out the name that you prefer, or are presently using. Being fully present in the moment, allow yourself to truly feel the vibrational energy in your name. Honor it. Celebrate it! Note the difference in your feelings, compared to what you felt during the release of the charged name(s).

Complete the exercise by using your current name within the following self empowering affirmation: "(Your Name), I unconditionally love, trust, and support you, just the way you are, in body, mind, and spirit, and in sound, light, and love." Repeat as needed.

Because individuals have their own unique experiences, results to this exercise may vary. You may have an extraordinary release and healing in doing the name toning process only once or twice, or, as with other release work, you may need to regularly return to the exercise and continue to chip away at old programming and feelings. Either way, your intent will dictate your results. I encourage periodic name toning until you feel completely clear and free of past issues. This simple exercise can be a fun and easy way to "own your tone" and better tune your signature frequency. Prize your name, and name your prize!

Group Name Toning Exercise

When name toning is performed in a group, the purpose is to unite the loving vibrations and healing intentions of many for the benefit and support of one. In other words, the whole is always greater than the sum of its parts. So when the vocal toning of one's name is directed to an individual with focused, loving support from a group of kindred spirits, the results can be quite magical.

> *When the vocal toning of one's name is directed to an individual with focused, loving support from a group of kindred spirits, the results can be quite magical.*

I've been using various forms of this toning exercise in my workshops for almost 20 years; I refer to it as the "Voice of the Soul." Several years ago, I was surprised and delighted to learn that a number of sound practitioners—including my friends Jonathan Goldman and his mentor, Sara Benson—use a similar group sounding process. I often notice how sound-workers seem to intuitively tune into the same universal energies and principles.

This group toning practice involves surrounding an individual within a circle of "toners," with the intention of lovingly sounding the name of the one in the center of the circle. The "receiver" may stand, sit, or lie down with eyes closed to best receive the healing sounds of his or her name, which are toned collectively by the group. The receiver may tone along with the group, or just remain silent and do nothing but receive the nurturing and healing tones. The toning may last for a couple of minutes or longer, or until the group feels intuitively complete. After a short period of silence, the receiver gets up and rejoins the group, and another member takes his/her place inside the circle to receive his/her healing sounds.

The Voice of the Soul can be a beautiful and sacred sound ceremony. Candles and incense can enhance the resonant ambience. What's most important is that everyone align with a loving intention to allow Divine Consciousness to be present. This group healing process can be very transformational, and great fun as well. Individuals who participate in this empowering group toning frequently report having beautiful visions, mystical experiences and profound healings.

≈

(((((10)))))

Chakra Chanting, Toning, and Balancing

If one ascends to the spiritual world...one can say that it consists entirely of vowels. Lacking the bodily instrument, one enters a tonal world colored in a variety of ways with vowels.

—Rudolf Steiner

A fun and popular toning practice involves using the vibrations of the vowels and voice to tone and align the chakras. Because we are vibrational beings, sound and toning can be far more effective methods for aligning the chakras than attempting to visualize these subtle energy centers of the body.

Chakras are not materially based, so they cannot be described from a purely physiological or materialistic standpoint. Just as a symphony cannot be described from the standpoint of musical notes and instruments or varying harmonics of sound—even though these can be said to form the basic structure of a symphony—similarly, the chakras cannot be described in terms of psychology, physiology, or any other physical science. Chakras are energy centers, or vital life force vortices within the human body, that are interrelated with the parasympathetic, sympathetic, and autonomous nervous systems.

Spinning Wheels

Chakra, a Sanskrit word, means "wheel," and denotes circle and movement. Essentially, the chakras are spinning wheels of energy. From another perspective, they can be thought of as "waves" of the mind that move in an "ocean of desires." And desires, as can waves, can direct energetic forces. Each chakra is a step-by-step plateau of desires containing and moving great vital force energies.

> *Desires, as can waves, can direct energetic forces.*

Throughout our lives we undulate in this ocean of desires, viewing and understanding life's vast array of activities and circumstances from the standpoint of the chakra in which we feel most comfortable.

East/West

Although most available information on chakras has been obtained from Hindu and Sanskrit traditions, it is by no means limited to Eastern thought. Many esoteric traditions and metaphysical practices have elaborated on these subtle energy centers of the body and their correlations to physical, emotional, mental, and spiritual well-being. Here in the West, in the last decade or more, there has been an increasing interest in the fields of sound therapy, vibrational healing, and subtle-energy medicine—including studies of their various components, such as chakra alignment and balancing.

In discussing the chakras we are necessarily discussing the subtle aspects of the energy centers in the body. The connection between the gross and subtle in the human organism is through intermediate conductors, or chakras, that are connected with the organs, particularly to the endocrine system. The chakras influence—and are influenced by—specific physical areas of the body (and corresponding emotions) where they are located. Various physical, emotional, and mental disharmonies and imbalances may be observed to be the results of imbalanced chakras.

Chakra Toning and Sonic Meditation

The two most effective ways of harmonizing and balancing the chakras are through chakra toning and sonic meditation.

Chakra toning is simply using specific tones or vowel sounds—along with proper breath support—to vocally direct vibrational energy into each chakra needing to be cleansed, aligned, and balanced. This chapter is devoted to exploring this methodology in great detail.

Sonic meditation is a subtler extension of this work, wherein the practitioner stills the mind and silently listens to the "inner sounds" for regeneration, equanimity, and peace. This transformational process not only supports the chakras but can also assist in mastering and transcending them as well. With continued application and practice, this spiritual discipline can aid the practitioner in achieving deeper states of consciousness and eventual ascension on the celestial Sound Current within. (This topic will be discussed later in this chapter.)

Note: Any closed-eye toning process—such as chakra toning—could be considered a preliminary form of sonic meditation.

Chakra Locations and Functions

Before discussing the principles and exercises involved in the process of tonal chakra balancing, let us first look at a brief description of each specific chakra, along with its location and functions within the body. In most esoteric teachings, reference is made to six or seven major chakras.

1. **Base or Root Chakra.**
   ≈ Located at the base of the spine, including the region between the anus and genitals and the first three vertebrae.
   ≈ Associated with the adrenal glands, overall circulation, gross physical body, issues of survival, order, structure, and groundedness.
   ≈ Often related visually to the color red, musically to the note of C, and to the element of Earth.
   ≈ Muladhara chakra in Sanskrit.

2. **Sacral Chakra.**
   ≈ Located below the navel, between and including the genitals and the hypogastric plexus.
   ≈ Associated with the sexual organs and reproductive system. Also relates to interactions between family and friends, including issues of security, intimacy, sexuality, personal boundaries, desires and attachments, primal emotions, and fantasy.
   ≈ Often related visually to the color orange, musically to the note of D, and to the element of Water.
   ≈ Svadhisthana chakra in Sanskrit.

3. **Solar Plexus or Navel Chakra.**
   ≈ Located 2 to 3 inches above the navel, including the solar plexus and the epigastric plexus.
   ≈ Associated with the digestive system. Also relates to self-esteem, identity, willpower, confidence, ego, practicality, responsibility, and organization.
   ≈ Often related visually to the color yellow, musically to the note of E, and to the element of Fire.
   ≈ Manipura chakra in Sanskrit.

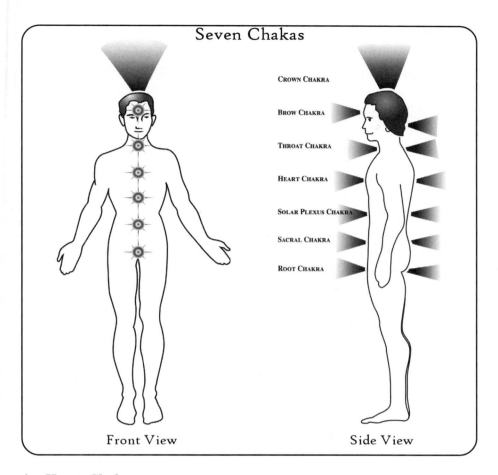

Seven Chakas

CROWN CHAKRA

BROW CHAKRA

THROAT CHAKRA

HEART CHAKRA

SOLAR PLEXUS CHAKRA

SACRAL CHAKRA

ROOT CHAKRA

Front View   Side View

4. **Heart Chakra.**

≈ Located at the cardiac plexus, in the center of the chest between the two nipples.

≈ Associated with the thymus gland, as well as the organs of the heart and respiratory system. Also relates to pure emotions of love, compassion, empathy, forgiveness, openness, authenticity, healing, and balance.

≈ Referred to as the "central" chakra, or "switching station," in the center of the body's vibrational matrix.

≈ Related visually to the color green, musically to the note of F or F-sharp (F♯), and to the element of Air.

≈ Anahata chakra in Sanskrit.

5. **Throat Chakra.**

   ≈ Located at the carotid plexus, or throat center.

   ≈ Associated with the thyroid gland. Also relates to speech, hearing, communication, creativity, teaching, and self-expression.

   ≈ Related visually to the color blue, musically to the note of G, and to the element of Ether or Akasha.

   ≈ Vishuddha chakra in Sanskrit.

6. **The Third Eye or Brow Chakra.**

   ≈ Located at the medulla plexus, pineal plexus, between the eyebrows—just above and behind the eyes.

   ≈ Associated with the pituitary and pineal glands. Also relates to imagination, intuition, insight, aspiration, spontaneity, psychic abilities, worldly detachment, truth, and wisdom.

   ≈ Often related visually to the colors indigo or purple, musically to the note A, and to the pure, rarefied essence of all elements.

   ≈ Ajna chakra in Sanskrit.

7. **Crown Chakra.**

   ≈ Supposedly located at the cerebral plexus, or top of the cranium. Actual location is within and beyond the crown of the head, but subtle aspects of this chakra can be perceived by some as glowing light, or a halo, as depicted in various pictures of saints and the spiritually enlightened.

   This inner chakra—and its many minor, or sub-chakras—cannot be fully accessed until the sixth chakra (third eye) is opened through spiritual practice, devotion, and grace. The seventh is often the most misunderstood chakra, due to its aspects frequently being taught incorrectly by those whose sixth chakra has not yet opened.

   ≈ Associated with enlightenment, illumination, spirituality, divinity, immortality, nothingness, transcendence, bliss, and Oneness. This chakra also relates to the "thousand-petal lotus," an umbrella-like arrangement of lotus petals that generates tremendous inner light from the astral universe/level of consciousness.

   This is one of the many wondrous, beautiful, and real experiences that lies within every human being and is accessible through spiritual devotion and meditation on the Sound Current.

≈ Often related visually to the color violet, and musically to the note B, the seventh chakra and various other inner chakras actually exist in an ascending, vibratory scale of sound, light, and pure Spirit—each subsequent, higher chakra emanating more brilliant light and celestial sound than the previous one. The seventh chakra is beyond individuated elements and relates to the "one element"— consisting of pure sound, light, and love: True Reality.

≈ Sahasrara chakra in Sanskrit.

Now that we have outlined the specific chakras and some of their relationships to the body, let us look at the ways in which we can use chakra toning to clear, balance, and revitalize these powerful energy centers.

Clarity of Intention

A number of books have been written about the chakras and their correlations to our overall well-being. Much of this information may be inconsistent and confusing to those who want to simply understand and use the most pertinent principles and effective exercises for chakra balancing and alignment. My intention in elaborating on various points of information described in this chapter is not to create further confusion in the readers, or to claim the best or only method of chakra alignment. Rather, I wish to offer a simple-to-use yet focused foundation for practical application. There are many methods for aligning the chakras. My suggested methods focus primarily on sound—specifically vocal sound, or toning—which is the quickest, easiest, and most effective modality for any chakra work.

Some individuals may be quite sensitive in feeling the sounds of the chakras—some even see them!—but it may take a little time and practice for others to feel confident and comfortable with the chakra toning process. By the second or third time doing the complete exercise, all of the components should fall into place and the chakra toning will feel very empowering and transformative.

Vowel Toning

The easiest yet most effective method for chakra clearing and balancing is *vowel toning*. Why vowel toning? Vowels are generally a universal language. Regardless of race, culture, country, or language, vowels in some form are always used by the voice. There may be more or less than the five vowels, and pronunciations might be slightly different from language to language. But all vowels open up the natural resonance of the voice more effectively than consonant sounds, or other non-vowel sounds. This allows the optimal energetic flow of prana to support the sound.

Note Toning

Another good reason for using vowel toning is that it doesn't require singing or musical training to master the process. It matters not if one is an accomplished singer or tone deaf—because it's not about aesthetic, tonal beauty or the use of a musical scale for singing specific notes.

Some systems of chakra balancing do use specific musical notes for each chakra, though there is often disagreement about the note correlations. Using simple vowel sounds tends to be more effective. As with most universal principles—the simplest is usually best.

This isn't to say that it is bad or wrong to work with the chakras using a musical note system—by all means follow your intuition and whatever works for you. I'm merely suggesting it's not likely that there is a universal requirement that you study music theory before attempting to tone your chakras.

Stepping Stones

One final, yet no less important, reason to use vowels in chakra toning is the way in which the vowels act as stepping stones in developing the voice's natural expression of overtones and harmonics. These multiple tones lie hidden within the various vowel sounds and give the voice its resonance. The development and conscious use of these vocal harmonics and overtones has been shown to have regenerative, as well as interdimensional, properties. This will be discussed further in Chapter 11.

Chakra Toning Preparation

As with most toning exercises, it is important to start with some preparatory steps before beginning the chakra toning process.

First, find a comfortable place to sit—in a chair, on a couch, or on the floor. You may sit cross-legged in the lotus position, or with your feet flat on the floor. Allow your whole body to be relaxed, but with your back reasonably straight. Close your eyes. Breathe deeply and diaphragmatically.

Next, practice any invocation or prayer that aligns you with Spirit. This will always enhance any toning exercise you do.

Now, begin the Resonant Breathing Exercise (described in Chapter 7). This step should take only about 90 seconds, once learned and practiced. Because this breathing exercise ends with the focus at the first chakra, your attention is precisely where it needs to be for beginning the Chakra Toning Exercise. You could also call this "chakra chanting" in an exercise form.

The Chakra Toning Exercise

It is necessary to give sufficient time to the vowel toning of each chakra. I usually recommend approximately two minutes each. It takes about this length of time for the chakra to respond and resonate. At times, you may feel a need to increase the time for a particular chakra. This is fine, but two minutes is usually sufficient.

Also important is noting your time intuitively, with intention, not by looking at your watch or clock. Keep your eyes closed, with your attention fixed within on the chakra. It's far better to be a few seconds off your time—remaining focused—than exactly on time but distracted and unfocused.

Because you'll be working with seven chakras, the entire length of time for the Chakra Toning Exercise should be approximately 15 minutes.

First Chakra

Begin by focusing your attention at the first (root) chakra, located at the base of the spine. While still breathing diaphragmatically, tone the "UH" vowel sound, as in the word *sun* or *fun*. Tone this sound at the deepest pitch you can comfortably make with your voice. Project the sound into the first chakra while holding your attention there. Tone this—and all other chakra vowels—in a soft to medium volume, without straining the voice.

Continue toning the "UH" vowel, pausing to breathe as needed, while sustaining the same low pitch for the full two minutes. (This is a vital point to fuse your frequency to the chakra for best results.) Don't allow your pitch to fluctuate. Find a comfortable pitch and sustain it.

During this toning time, hold your intention to align, cleanse, resonate, revitalize, and balance this chakra. Feel your energetic connection to the first chakra and notice if any particular feelings surface. Also, notice if you begin to visualize a particular color. Be aware if the "UH" vowel feels appropriate, or needs to change to a different vowel sound. If the "UH" sound feels comfortable to you, sustain your tonal focus on it.

Pitch

When you feel complete with "vowel-onating" the first chakra, begin to slowly raise the pitch of your voice, while simultaneously visualizing the energy rising upwards, from the first to the second chakra. Taking five to 10 seconds to raise your pitch between chakras is usually sufficient. This vocal pitch raising is an essential component of effective chakra toning, and should always be done between each chakra. It is a vital step in moving the energy properly for activating the chakras and in sensitizing your vibrational awareness.

A note of caution: Do not start with a first chakra pitch/note that is so high that, by the time you reach the sixth or seventh chakra, you have no vocal range left. This will defeat your purpose, and may strain your voice as well. Start low enough in pitch to give yourself ample pitch room.

As mentioned earlier, it may take practicing two or three times to intuitively and energetically determine the best pitch for your voice and each chakra. You'll find, however, by trusting in the sound and the process, that it's easier than you think. In fact, this is the only segment of the exercise that requires you to rely completely on your intuition to move more deeply into your chakras and your signature frequency. This in turn enhances your intuition for a more integrative and transformative experience.

Second Chakra

Upon finding the appropriate pitch for the second (sacral) chakra, shift your voice from the "UH" vowel, to the "OO" vowel sound, as in the word *food* or *true*. While focusing your attention at the second chakra point below the navel, project the sound softly but clearly into this area. The eyes should remain closed (throughout the entire exercise) as you continue breathing diaphragmatically, while sustaining the vowel and pitch for this chakra.

As with the first chakra, notice any movement of energy and any feelings that arise. It might be helpful to place your hands on the chakra area for added connection and focus. Feel the sound and vibrational energy expand, gradually resonating and filling your whole body. Be aware of any light or colors that you may visualize. Listen and feel if the "OO" vowel needs to shift to another sound. While remaining fully present in the moment, continue toning the second chakra for two minutes or so.

When you feel complete with aligning and balancing the second chakra, begin to raise your vocal pitch—as with the previous chakra—to discover the right pitch and location for toning the third chakra.

Third Chakra

Upon finding an appropriately higher pitch for the third (navel) chakra at the solar plexus area, shift your voice from the "OO" vowel to the "OH" vowel sound, as in the word *no* or *toe*. While focusing your attention on this chakra, project the "OH" sound there, while sustaining your pitch, in the same manner as the previous chakra. Again, notice any shifts in your energy, feelings, and visualizations, and anything else you may experience.

As you feel the energy of the third chakra begin to expand and resonate throughout your entire body, allow it to guide you through any other vowel sounds you may feel—or simply continue toning the "OH" sound. After two minutes—or when you feel complete with toning and balancing the third chakra—begin raising your vocal pitch to locate the next chakra.

Fourth Chakra

Upon elevating your pitch and visualization to the fourth (heart) chakra, shift your vocal toning from the "OH" vowel to the "AH" vowel sound, as in the word *drama* or *chakra*. Focusing your attention at the heart chakra in the center of the chest (not on the physical heart, which is to the left of center), project the "AH" sound—softly and gently—into this area.

Follow the same method and guidelines as the previous chakras, while sustaining the vocal pitch you've selected for the fourth chakra. Continue breathing diaphragmatically with eyes closed, remaining relaxed but holding your intention to align, clear, and balance your fourth chakra. Resonate this "heart center" by toning the "AH" vowel for the next couple of minutes.

Upon feeling complete with the heart chakra resonation, begin raising your pitch from the vocal midrange of the heart chakra, to a slightly higher pitch, conducive to connecting with the throat chakra.

The Switching Station

The fourth chakra, or heart center, is often referred to as the "switching station," as it is the chakra centerpoint in the body.

In teaching various toning practices such as ***tantra toning*** (see Chapter 15) and targeted chakra work, I often recommend starting at the heart center because, for many, it's easier to tone and access this chakra in place of beginning with the first or second chakra. For one reason, it's more natural and comfortable for the voice to be in the middle vocal range for most people. Secondly, because the heart chakra rules love, compassion, and healing, it's a good and useful starting point for more easily accessing one's real vibrational energy. From this switching station, you may move up or down the chakras, as needed.

This approach, however, should not be seen as a shortcut to avoid working with the first three chakras. It is primarily recommended as an alternative access point, if there is any difficulty in beginning at the first chakra, or when one is desirous of concentrating on healing one or two specific chakras. This is usually more successful after sufficient experience has been gained by learning and regularly practicing the complete chakra toning exercise, as outlined here.

Fifth Chakra

The optimal vowel sound for toning the fifth (throat) chakra is the "AY" sound, as in the word *say* or *play*. With focused attention, project this toning sound into the fifth chakra, while sustaining the appropriate vocal pitch. Again, follow all the necessary steps outlined for the previous chakras.

Although no more or less important than the other chakras, added significance may be assigned to the fifth chakra in that it rules communication, creative self-expression, and, of course, toning.

Upon completing the fifth chakra toning and balancing, allow your intuition to guide you in lifting your vocal pitch and visualization to the next chakra, above and behind the eyes.

Sixth Chakra

After a satisfactorily higher pitch has been reached for the sixth (brow) chakra, change your vowel to the "EE" sound, as in the word *see* or *free*. This vowel sound works best with the sixth chakra, also referred to as the third eye.

While sustaining your vocal pitch, with a clear intention, complete the necessary steps described in the previous chakra points for toning and balancing the sixth chakra.

As this chakra rules intuition and higher knowledge, you may feel energized and inspired by a kind of natural knowingness or psychic momentum that may enhance your awareness. It is important, however, to remain focused in your attention while toning this third-eye chakra for the best results.

Seventh Chakra

Upon completing the sixth chakra toning, it is now time to bring the pitch and attention up to the final, seventh (crown) chakra. As with the sixth chakra, the vowel sound for toning and aligning the seventh chakra is also the "EE" vowel. The only aspects that are different, at this point, are the pitch of the voice and the focus of the attention.

> *The "real" spiritual journey begins at the third eye—and ascends inward and upward from there.*

Your pitch should move up to the highest note that your voice can comfortably project. The attention should be focused a few inches above the crown of the head. Again, following the toning guidelines of all the previous chakras, sustain this high-pitched "EE" vowel sound for at least two minutes, or until you feel intuitively complete. Then be silent and in the moment.

Crown Controversy

As indicated in the section on "Chakra Locations and Functions," it is important to remember that the crown chakra may be truly accessed only after the third eye has been opened at the sixth chakra. There has been confusion and controversy regarding this point, particularly here in the West. However, the Masters of the Sound Current (spiritual adepts who are experienced in traversing the inner realms of higher consciousness with Sacred Sound) tell us that the real spiritual journey begins at the third eye—and ascends inward and upward from there.

As the attention collects and concentrates at the third-eye center, gradually the third eye—or "single eye," as it is sometimes referred to—begins to *flutter* open, and then close. Eventually, with practice, discipline, and spiritual devotion, it remains open. Only then will one be able to enter the glorious inner realms of the seventh chakra—and beyond—that lie within each and every one of us. Regions of indescribable beauty and light are then experienced, including the magnificent "thousand-petal lotus" described by the mystics.

Sonic Meditation

After completing the entire Chakra Toning Exercise, it is not unusual to feel quite euphoric, to hear inner sounds, or to enter into an altered state of consciousness. Do not be alarmed; you will likely feel only peaceful. This is the state of *sonic meditation*. In this state, you may hear celestial sounds, or even the Inner Overtone or Sacred Sound Current. This sound or sonic meditation is the purest form of meditation because it unites us with the Divine and will eventually carry us to our True Home on its Current.

It is quite appropriate and very beneficial to sit silently in this state. Your focused attention will become more concentrated, and this is essential for productive meditation. You will be better able to still the overactive "monkey" mind. Trust yourself and your process. Relax and enjoy the rewards of aligned chakras and expanded inner awareness.

Sit quietly focused within after most toning exercises, as it greatly assists in accelerating spiritual development. You will then be on the threshold to opening the inner chakras and accessing the infinite wonders of the Sound Current—your true heritage.

Grounding

The final step in the Chakra Toning Exercise, and the sonic meditation process, is to fully ground oneself in the body. This usually takes only 15 to 30 seconds, and it greatly assists in the grounding necessary for returning to one's daily activities and responsibilities.

To easily accomplish this, focus your attention at the crown of the head and take in a deep, diaphragmatic breath. Release the breath through the mouth, while toning the "EE" vowel sound—the last toning vowel used. As you release the sound, "ride" your voice down in pitch while simultaneously visualizing your attention moving from the crown down through the chakras.

Riding Down Sound

Bring your attention down, past the brow, past the throat to the heart center, and pause. Take a second deep breath at this switching station and continue to move down in your visualization and pitch, as you now shift to the "AH" vowel sound.

Keep coming down, past the heart center, past the solar plexus—further down—past the abdomen, all the while moving deeper in your pitch, until reaching the first chakra point at the base of the spine. Allow your voice to subtly shift from the "AH" to the lowest "UH" sound you can make, while releasing any remaining air from your lungs.

Upon bringing your attention to the root chakra—while releasing all breath and sound—feel your total connection with your physical body temple. Then slowly open your eyes, take a deep breath, stretch your body as needed, and allow yourself to feel energized and revitalized, yet fully present, completely grounded, relaxed, at peace, and, above all, truly grateful for your experience.

This is a simple, fast, and excellent way to ground yourself after any deep toning process or meditation. I suggest using it often, as needed.

≈

Gender Energy

Oftentimes, a strong or weak *gender energy* may influence your chakras. Gender energy refers to your male or female energy. Being self-aware of any strengths and weaknesses in your voice can be useful in identifying any issues or energy imbalances related to your gender. And some simple chakra "tone-tweaking" may assist you in correcting them.

For example, women seldom use the lower range of their voices, as men usually do, and may have some resistance or difficulty in doing so. The results of not using the lower voice often are a weak first—and sometimes second—chakra. This may indicate a lack of "male energy" attributes, such as groundedness, assertiveness, or self power.

This can be compensated for and corrected by spending some additional time in toning the first two chakras. An extra minute or two each during the chakra toning exercise is usually sufficient. This same advice applies to men who speak with a high-pitched voice in the upper vocal register, and may have an overabundance of "female energy."

Chakra-Challenged

Most men tend to be more comfortable using their deeper, more masculine "chest voice." They often have resistance and difficulty accessing and using their falsetto, or "head voice." This is due, at least in part, to repressive societal programming and fear of exhibiting their feminine side. As a result, men frequently find it challenging to express their full vocal range, emotions, and innate female energy.

Though generally more grounded and stronger in their first and second chakras, men tend to be weaker—if not blocked altogether—in the upper chakras. After all, that well-worn cliché is never referred to as "men's intuition."

With chakra toning, however, these blockages can be easily overcome. I suggest that men—or women with a lot of male energy—spend some additional time in toning their upper chakras. An extra minute or two in toning both the sixth and seventh chakras is usually sufficient—or until you feel vocally and "chakrally" integrated.

Damage Control

I must emphasize a very important point here: Never push the voice beyond its natural limits. Although you should always be in your upper vocal range while toning the higher chakras, don't overextend your range or volume. This is unnecessary for effective chakra toning and may damage your voice.

Target Chakras

As mentioned in the fourth chakra/switching station section, it is sometimes useful to target and tone individual chakras. There may be occasions when you feel only one or two chakras are out of balance and affecting the others, or that only certain emotions are being stressed—for example, an inability to be sexually or emotionally intimate (second chakra), low confidence or self-esteem (third chakra), or difficulty with giving and receiving love (fourth chakra). In these cases, you may want to focus your toning practice on those chakras pertinent to the stress. This can be most helpful, particularly in time-sensitive circumstances, when it may not be appropriate or possible to do the complete chakra toning exercise.

For instance, I recall a time when I was running late en route to a lecture I was to present. I hadn't had sufficient time to tone and meditate that day, so I was somewhat out of sorts. Also, being unfamiliar with the group I was to speak to and the location of the event further added to my stress.

While driving to my destination, I decided that I needed to take advantage of the drive time to tone the appropriate chakras. I began with a silent invocation, and then proceeded to tone the "AH" vowel to resonate my heart chakra, which felt shut down due to my judgments toward myself and others. (Of course, I kept my eyes open during this process, as I was driving and needed no further complications!)

Chakra Traffic

I projected the sound into my fourth chakra with the intention to open love and compassion toward myself and others (including any rude drivers). After sustaining the vowel toning for approximately six to eight minutes I began feeling more open, loving, and accepting of myself, and a greater awareness of the perfection of divine circumstances. I blessed and released the energy I had perceived to be immobilizing me.

Then I shifted my attention to the throat center, and began toning the "AY" sound into my fifth chakra. Recognizing that, in order to fully express my creative self and voice my soul, I needed to resonate and balance this chakra. After sounding the "AY" vowel for about eight to 10 minutes, with the intention of opening my voice and expressing my spirit, I felt complete.

Clear "AH"-Rival

I arrived at the conference feeling clear, fully centered, aligned with spirit, and inspired to give my presentation.

Having derived great benefits from the use of these toning tools, I often feel grateful for these uplifting experiences. I invite you to do the same, and support you in developing, using, and enjoying your chakra tones.

Chakra Combinations

Allow your energy and intuition to assist you in identifying any chakra, or combinations of chakras, in need of balancing and toning work. In one instance, it may be two or three chakras needing alignment. In another, perhaps, it's only one chakra—such as the third, which relates to self-esteem and ego issues.

Any time you feel it's appropriate, target and focus your toning on the particular chakra(s) in need of balancing. Between five and 10 minutes each is usually sufficient.

Chakra Chanting

In 1995, I had a unique and empowering experience while camping at the foot of Mt. Rainier in the state of Washington. During my morning meditation, a particular melody—accompanied by a series of vowel sounds—kept running through my head. As I continued to tone these sounds while shaving, I realized the Chakra Chant had birthed itself.

Though it's not a substitute for the Chakra Toning Exercise, I have used this fun and simple Chakra Chant in my seminars for many years as a means for immediate chakra stimulation. (The Chakra Chant is also included on my second healing music CD, *In Chantment.*)

The Chakra Chant

"UH-OO-OH-AH-AY-EE" (4x)

"AH-EE-AY"

"AH-EE-OH"   Bridge/Turnaround

"AH-EE"

"UH-OO-OH-AH-AY-EE" (Repeat as above)

Key:

"UH"   (1st chakra)

"OO"   (2nd chakra)

"OH"   (3rd chakra)

"AH"   (4th chakra)

"AY"   (5th chakra)

"EE"   (6th and 7th chakras)

Intention:

"UH-OO-OH-AH-AY-EE"

Designed to align and empower all chakras.

"AH-EE-AY"

Send unconditional love and empowerment to others (via the 5th chakra).

"AH-EE-OH"

Bring the energy back to support oneself (3rd chakra).

"AH-EE"

Focus the heart to continue the chakra cycle (4th chakra).

(To facilitate better concentration of the energy, place the palms of the hands at each corresponding chakra while going through the chant.)

≈

Various Systems

Over the last several years, toning has increased in popularity as a self-supportive, expressive, and transformative process. Along with this development, various systems of toning the chakras with vowels have emerged. Although most of these systems are inherently similar and generally useful, they may tend to lock one into certain sounds, or vowels, without factoring in the individual's signature frequency and sonic intuition. This type of approach to toning doesn't look at the bigger picture, or fully empower the individual.

On one hand, we don't want to ignore or throw out the research and experience of others. Yet, at the same time, we need to stay in the moment, and trust in ourselves and the development of our vibratory awareness.

Sonic Suggestions

In this light, I have a few suggestions: First, recognize that the clarity of your intention is just as important as the type of sound you use. This is why various systems of chakra toning that seem to be in conflict with each other may still prove to be effective. So, begin with a clear intention regarding the results you want to achieve from your chakra toning.

Secondly, select a vowel system that makes sense to you as a logical chakra toning foundation. In most types of toning exercises, the best results can be gained by beginning with a clear, focused, and pragmatic approach.

> *The clarity of your intention is just as important as the type of sound you use.*

Next, try to set aside any fixed or rigid attitudes you may be holding, and tune into your sense of spontaneity and intuition. Trust in your higher self and the expression of its sound. Then, sensitize yourself to the particular chakra you're toning and allow yourself to be guided by the designated vowel—or whatever sound feels intuitively correct, in the moment—for that chakra.

Lastly, remember that the most effective attitude toward toning practices is one that embraces flexibility, creativity, and gratefulness.

Tones are never set in stone.

Tonal Tips

For the best results with chakra toning, I recommend the following:

≈   In the morning upon arising, tone the Siren Vowel Exercise (page 65) for about five minutes, or until your voice is properly warmed up. A great time for this may be in the shower or while dressing.

≈ Find a comfortable place to sit, close your eyes, and silently say a prayer or invocation for establishing a spiritual environment, while breathing deeply and diaphragmatically.

≈ After feeling focused and connected with your spirit, begin the 90-second Resonant Breathing Exercise (page 68). Upon completion, your attention will be on the first chakra, at the base of the spine.

≈ Using the appropriate vowel sounds—and sustaining your vocal pitch—tone and balance each chakra for two minutes.

≈ To clear and uplift the energy, raise your vocal pitch between each successive chakra.

≈ After the chakra toning and balancing is complete, sit in silent meditation for as long as convenient, remaining receptive and fully present.

≈ Upon feeling intuitively complete with your chakra balancing and meditative experience, begin the grounding process for returning to your outer body awareness.

≈ If at times you are unable to do the complete Chakra Toning Exercise (page 93), you may focus attention on toning the chakra(s) in need of the most support.

≈ Use the benefits of your chakra toning to consistently create a joyous and transformative experience. Always complete your toning exercises by fully offering gratitude to the Infinite Loving Spirit within you for the gift of your experience.

Although these techniques and suggestions are very specific, they are not meant to be rigid or all-encompassing. Each person has his/her own unique experience and signature frequency to add to the mix. Openness and flexibility harmonize your soul.

Openness and flexibility harmonize your soul.

Most importantly, you use your self-awareness and intuition to guide you. Notice if you have any fear or resistance in any chakra, or within any part of your vocal register. If so, spend sufficient time toning there, until the energy opens and shifts—until you feel resonance and harmony. This is one of the inherent principles of toning.

Chakra Blues
(The End of the Blues)

We can't change anybody
'Cause everybody gets to choose.
But if we choose to heal ourselves
It'll be the end of the blues.
The spread of hate and fear—
they dominate the news.
It's time to walk our talk of love
to the end of the blues.
We can rise up through the chakras
Seeing all the vibrant hues,
From the reds and greens and violets,
to the end of the blues.
Doubt and limitation
is all we have to lose.
There's infinity of freedom
At the end of the blues.
Now, it's time to journey homeward
To those wondrous inner views.
Seeing sound and hearing light,
Awakening souls enjoy the cruise—
Where the drop becomes the ocean
At the end of the blues.
The end of the blues.

—Wayne Perry

(((((11)))))

Overtoning: A Sonic Harmonic Tonic

*The voice is not only audible, but also visible, to those
who can see it; the voice makes impressions on the
ethereal spheres, impressions which can be called audible
but are visible at the same time.*

*On all planes the voice makes an impression, and those
scientists who have made experiments with sound and have
taken impressions of sound on plates will find one day that
the impression of the voice is more living, more deep, and
has a greater effect than any other sound.*

—Hazrat Inayat Khan

When light passes through a crystal or prism, a beautiful rainbow of
colors is projected onto most any surface. Similarly, when sound passes
through a chamber—whether a cave, horn, or guitar body—a beautiful
spectrum of overtones and harmonics can be heard. And likewise, by projecting vocal sounds through the various chambers of the human body—
particularly the oral, throat, and nasal cavities—extraordinary vocal
harmonics and overtones can be created, heard, and felt.

Overtoning is the vocal practice of sounding two or more tones simultaneously. The technique of overtoning involves modulating the resonant
cavities in the head and throat to make audible combinations of partial
tones, while at the same time sounding a lower fundamental tone. Though
not easily heard when they are not emphasized, the overtones are the component parts of the fundamental note being toned.

The creation of overtones may be better facilitated by manipulating
the oral chamber, tongue, lips, jaw, pharynx, and nasal cavities, while
alternating between different pitches. The development of this technique
can produce remarkable, angelic, otherworldly, whistling, and bell-like
sounds, which at times seem to be emanating from various directions.

Although there are some in the toning community who make a distinction that overtoning is a specific diagnostic or scanning technique, in fact, overtoning is simply a general term for the process of creating vocal overtones and harmonics. This process may be used in a number of ways, as we will discuss throughout this and other chapters.

Sonic Bouquets

Multiple tones or harmonics are naturally present in everyone's speaking and singing voice. We generally don't hear them because of the relative rapidity of the normal vocal pattern, and because we tend to focus on the words or message being conveyed. However, when we slow down the articulation of the voice and emphasize certain vowel sounds and consonants, the harmonics and overtones begin to emerge and can be more easily heard.

The practice of overtoning requires the opposite approach to how a good diction or singing teacher might instruct a student in achieving the best voice control. Most teachers, for example, would emphasize a clear distinction between each vowel sound for clear enunciation, whereas the best way to allow the harmonics to emerge is by "slurring," merging, and elongating the vowels—slowly running them together. This technique enables the voice to evoke sonic bouquets of blossoming harmonics.

While discussing vocal overtones in *The Book of Sound Therapy*, Olivea Dewhurst-Maddock writes:

> It is helpful to picture them as the petals of a flower, closed and folded inward. Overtone chanting aims to open the flower and reveal the true beauty, complexity and delicacy of the bloom. It is truly amazing to hear the constituent elements of the voice opened out, clearly and separately, with the sets of overtones being produced simultaneously.

Harmonics and Overtones

Actually quantum in nature, harmonics and overtones are geometric multiples created by the specific frequency of an object. Because everything is composed of frequency and vibration, everything creates overtones and harmonics. The overtones determine the character and quality of the individual sounds that we hear. Though we may not be able to distinguish each overtone that makes up a particular sound, the overtones shape the texture, timbre, and overall color of the sound, giving an instrument or voice its uniqueness.

These distinctive clusters of overtones and harmonics, where the vibrational energy of the sound is most concentrated, are sometimes referred to as "formants."

There may be some confusion about whether there is a difference between harmonics and overtones, particularly among those untrained musically. For all intents and purposes they are the same. However, from another perspective it may be useful to define a difference between them.

Fundamentals

It is important to first recognize that every tone or note contains within it all other tones and notes. Think about this. For example, although we may not be able to see it, within the seed is the flower. Within the acorn is the oak tree. Within the human body is the soul—Infinite Spirit. Similarly, although we may not be able to hear all of them, a countless array of overtones is vibrating within any single, fundamental note.

> *Every tone or note contains within it all other tones and notes.*

A frequency of 256 Hz, for instance, vibrates in the range of the musical note C. We may call this its fundamental tone, and it is the predominant sound that we hear. Within this frequency or note of C, however, numerous other notes are sounding in addition to the fundamental tone. These are referred to as overtones. In musical parlance they are synonymously called harmonics.

Each ascending octave of C that is vibrating within this fundamental note represents an overtone, and vibrates at exactly twice the number of cycles per second as the previous note. (Example: 512 Hz—second octave of C; 1024 Hz—the third octave; 2048 Hz—fourth octave; 4096 Hz—fifth octave; and so on.) However, within these octaves, numerous other tones and notes are sounded that are harmonic counterparts to the fundamental note of C and its ascending octaves. These tones may be referred to as harmonics, for they represent a complementary tonal color or harmony.

Every harmonic is considered an overtone as well, because it has a higher frequency than the fundamental and represents an additional tone. Every overtone, however, is not necessarily a harmonic from this perspective, because "octave overtones" do not create a musical harmony with the fundamental.

Musical Relationship

In musical terminology, the **overtone series** indicates that overtones are mathematically related to each other. These relationships can have profound effects upon the harmonious and healing aspects of sound. In the practice of sound therapy, the regenerative power of overtones can play an important role in establishing body-mind harmony. And from a spiritual perspective, the ascending overtone series represents evolution and its relationship to the Infinite Sound Current, which creates and sustains all frequencies of beingness.

The following diagram, which I call the Overtone Spiral, illustrates and symbolizes some of the aspects of these relationships.

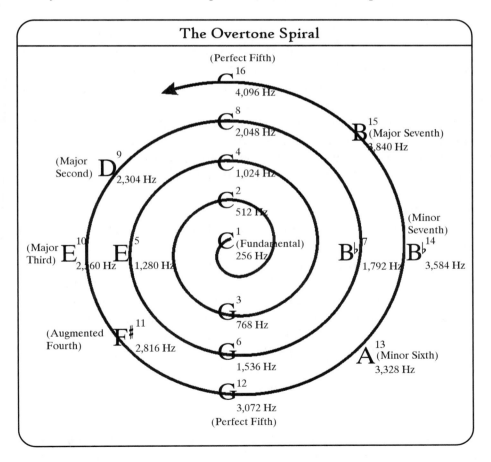

The Overtone Spiral

Using the note of C as the fundamental, it also shows the acorn effect discussed earlier, indicating the way every frequency/note is contained within any other given note. (The same harmonic ratios will arise regardless of the fundamental tone that is vibrated; however, different pitches are created depending upon the fundamental.)

The Overtone Spiral indicates the 16 notes of the first four octaves (vibrating at above 4,000 Hz) created by the harmonics of toning or striking the fundamental note of C. This is not, however, the completion of the overtones being created, as each ascending overtone, being a geometric multiple of the fundamental, vibrates at faster and higher frequencies, or cycles per second. We can potentially hear all of these notes/tones/frequencies until they reach about 20,000 Hz, after which—continuing to multiply—they vibrate beyond the human hearing range, ultimately, into infinity.

> *Sound never ends; it simply vibrates outside of our awareness.*

Sound never ends; it simply vibrates outside of our awareness. (At least until we reach total awareness!) This may relate to the sound reportedly heard by those revived from near-death experiences, who frequently claim to have heard beautiful, choir-like music or celestial harmony. Similarly, upon hearing vocal harmonics for the first time, many experience the sound as the "singing of angels."

Color My World

In a 1986 workshop in Toronto, David Hykes of the Harmonic Choir stated:

> The voice is like a person's signature or pulse—it says a lot about that person. It is like that refracted starlight whose colors reveal its elemental nature.... It is like the color spectrum: a few colors like red, orange, and yellow make all the marvelous, unique things we see. The same is true for sounds. There is only the harmonic series, and the whole sonic universe—if not Creation as a whole—comes out of that.

Harmony

Harmony is the foundation for all healing. The word *harmony* comes from the Greek root "harmos"—to fit together. When we allow ourselves to fit, join, or resonate with something, we bring ourselves into harmony with it. The inner experience of this harmony brings to us a deeper awareness of our fundamental or signature frequency.

> *Harmony is the foundation for all healing.*

Within the Inner Overtone or Sacred Sound Current, the fundamental is not a particular tone, note, or octave, as it is in music. The fundamental is all-pervading—existing in every dimension, every vibration, everything, including and especially ourselves. The ultimate healing involves returning to the Fundamental. But we cannot find it. Rather, the Fundamental is revealed to us as we allow ourselves to open, listen, resonate, and give voice to our souls. Then we will experience real freedom, inner peace, and true harmony.

> *The ultimate healing involves returning to the Fundamental.*

Creating Harmonics

The head of the Sufi Order in the West, Pir Vilayat Khan has said, "The true healing power of sound comes from the chanting of harmonics." These wondrous yet innate vocal sounds can be a vehicle for accessing the inner portals, helixes, and grid points within the mind-body that lead us to accelerated healing and expanded human awareness. In her Pleiadian book, *Bringers of the Dawn*, Barbara Marciniak writes, "When you create harmonics of sound, it reminds your body of something. It reminds your body of light, of deep cosmic love, and of other worlds."

The harmonics can also regenerate, repattern, align, and tune the frequencies of the body, while at the same time they are fun to make and intriguing to listen to. Discovering and sounding the harmonics and overtones in your voice requires no formal singing or musical training, and is indeed a joyful, enriching, and transformative experience.

It has been postulated that these extraordinary vocal sounds have tremendous healing power and can massage the body from the inside out. Just as an opera singer may shatter a crystal wine glass by producing a high, sustained tone, similarly, the power of vocal overtones can shatter subtle energy blockages in the body, which can cause tension, stress, and pain, and may lead to disease.

Marciniak further states, "These harmonics can be utilized in incredible ways, for harmonics can evolve many things.... The harmonics alter something; they open the door. Certain combinations of sounds played through the human body unlock information and frequencies of intelligence."

Listening

Before we can use harmonics, it is vital that we learn to listen. As David Hykes stated at the 1986 workshop: "The harmonic can be a messenger. This becomes magical, because our world, like music, is a vibratory world. Our picture of it has to do with the way our listening or consciousness has crystallized it in us. We see only a kind of frozen architecture of listening."

Because experts in sound research have shown that all the sounds we make are based entirely on all the sounds we hear, the first step in learning to successfully create vocal harmonics is to listen to the harmonics. Just as speakers' and singers' voices take on the vocal inflections and characteristics of the voices that they listen to most, similarly, the more we listen to vocal harmonics, the more harmonic resonance will be exhibited in our voices. But this is only part of the benefit of listening to vocal harmonics.

> *All the sounds we make are based entirely on all the sounds we hear.*

There are even greater benefits to be had from listening to harmonics, as they can entrain and teach the brain to reproduce and strengthen weakened frequencies for therapeutic results. Regular listening to these harmonics—particularly in the pitches conducive to one's signature frequency—can be quite healing and regenerative.

Sound Therapy

When you compare the voice with the instrument, there is no real comparison, because the voice itself is alive. The movement, the glance, the touch, even the breath that come from the nostrils do not reach as far as the voice reaches.

—Hazrat Inayat Khan

During the first two years of my sound therapy practice when I was experimenting with tone generators, I would create various combinations of multiple frequencies for my clients to listen to. The purpose of this form of sound therapy was to first identify the missing tones evidenced in a client's voice, and then play back those tones to the client with the sound machine. Upon regular and repeated listening to multiple tones, the brain will entrain with them and restore its missing tones. (See Chapter 16.) This process is designed to correct the associated vibrational imbalances that can lead to disharmony and illness.

I subsequently learned that the sound machine I was using was simply mimicking the complex waveform patterns of harmonics in the human voice. Other than this, the machine differed little from other tone generators and sound machines. After this discovery (and others), I abandoned the use of sound machines and concentrated my practice exclusively on the use of natural vocal harmonics for sound healing.

Although there are various types of vocal toning that may be used therapeutically, in my experience, the appropriate use of vocal harmonics is the most powerful and effective. (See Chapter 20.) These magical sounds have an unlimited potential for moving, shaping, and transforming energy.

Why is this so? No one really knows for sure, but it may in part be due to the waveforms that are created by simultaneous, multiple tones, and the way the body receives them. Add to this the voice's direct connection to the "toner" and object of the toning, thereby eliminating the outer instrument, or middle-man, so to speak. Or, perhaps, as spiritual beings residing in physical bodies, we are simply gifted with the ability, or grace, to open the voice as a vehicle for Spirit and its transcendent sound, light, and love. One thing is certain: No instrument or machine has a soul or possesses this capacity.

Multiple Tones

One of the remarkable aspects of the overtoning process is its creation of multiple, combination, and difference tones. These multiple frequencies can expand and enhance vibrational healing potentials. For example, when overtoning creates two tones or notes, two additional tones (four total) are automatically created. To better understand this principle, let's suppose the first tone vibrates at 200 Hz and the second at 250 Hz. You will simultaneously get a third (combination) tone at 450 Hz (200 plus 250 Hz), and a fourth (difference) tone at 50 Hz (250 minus 200 Hz). This demonstrates how to create a multiple of four simultaneous frequencies with vocal harmonics and overtoning.

Shift Happens

In his book, *Shifting Frequencies*, my colleague Jonathan Goldman states, "Vocal harmonics can be an extraordinary means of heightening your consciousness. It changes your brainwaves and stimulates portions of your brain that can receive greater levels of frequency." Research has shown that many benefits may be gained by simply listening to vocal harmonics and overtones. Some of these benefits include:

≈ Reducing and relieving stress.

≈ Enhancing memory.

≈ Charging the cortex of the brain.

≈ Growing new brain cells.

≈ Teaching and entraining the brain to restore and replace weak, dormant, or missing frequencies.

≈ Stimulating and enhancing the functions of the immune system.

≈ Slowing down respiration, heartbeat, and brainwave activity.

≈ Improving the flow and pulse of cerebral spinal fluid.

≈ Creating new neural synaptic connections.

≈ Regenerating body systems.

≈ Expanding consciousness and inner awareness.

These states have occurred only by listening to vocal harmonics, not making them. Goldman goes on to say, "Sounds rich in harmonics nourish the body, brain and psyche. Simply by listening to the sounds you can learn to shift your frequencies." The more conscious and active your listening efforts are, the greater the benefits received from the harmonics. Similarly, when creating vocal harmonics and overtones, conscious intent combined with active participation will glean the best results and lead you to the incredible healing potentials of harmonics.

Food for Thought

If great benefits can be achieved by simply listening to harmonics, imagine the value of resonating one's own body with harmonics. This may be likened to the benefits derived from food: We may eat the most healthy and nutritious foods, but if we don't eliminate their by-products from the body we will develop a serious health problem. Similarly, we may eliminate

> *The more conscious and active your listening efforts are, the greater the benefits received from the harmonics.*

well, but if we don't eat enough nutritious foods we'll have health problems. What comes out is equally important as what goes into the body; it's a reciprocal flow of energy.

In much the same way, we may benefit by listening to healthy frequencies such as toning sounds or music created with vocal harmonics and overtones. But to derive the optimal benefits we need to also make these healthy sounds. In the next chapter we will unlock the "Secrets to Vocal Overtoning."

(((((12)))))

The Secrets to Vocal Overtoning

When we know the Overtone we know the secret of life.

—Wayne Perry

After listening to vocal sounds rich in harmonics, the next step is to prepare your body and vocal instrument to create overtones and harmonics. By making these wondrous tones you will experience deeper and more profound levels of receptivity, resonance, and regeneration.

After years of research, study, and experience in the fields of toning and sound therapy, I have found no better technique for successfully effecting healing and transformation than overtoning. During this time, I have taught this extraordinary vocal technique to many—young and old—throughout the United States and abroad, with gratifying results. I subsequently made a recording of 20 specific exercises (*The Secrets to Vocal Overtoning*) for home practice and for those unable to attend my workshops.

This process of creating two or more tones simultaneously with the voice is the most organically natural form of sound healing that I'm aware of. And it requires no formal voice training or singing experience—only intent and practice. All that is necessary to learn this fun and fascinating process is an open attitude, a willingness to practice, and patience with yourself.

Hands-On Hearing

The following practice will assist you in using "resonant listening" to better hear your own overtones: Hold one hand in a cupped position with your fingers together and halfway flexed, thumb against forefinger. Place this hand around and behind your outer ear as if you are straining to hear someone speaking in a noisy room. Make sure your fingers are closed with the hand half open, and not covering the ear canal, to assist the ear in collecting more sound.

While doing this, take the other hand and place it a few inches in front of your mouth with the palm toward you, fingers together and fully extended. This hand will act as a sounding board and allow the sound to reflect back to your ear. You may adjust the distance of your hand closer to or further from your mouth as needed to better hear the overtones. Again, remember to keep the fingers closed, or you will lose some of the reflected sound.

You now have an easy and convenient listening tool to assist you in hearing the overtones in your voice while practicing the upcoming exercises in this chapter. This can be particularly useful if there are distracting sounds in your environment or if, for any reason, you have difficulty hearing yourself. This method may also be used with any other toning exercise.

Vowels and Energy

Many overtones may be evoked through and between the vowels while toning. The vowels are the single most powerful sonic tool we have, because when resonated they produce the most sound by activating the most breath or prana. The consonants partially block or alter the sound and energy. In a scream, for example, we can create the maximum volume and energy with vowels. However, with overtoning it should be noted that our concern is with energy, not volume, as too much volume is unnecessary and can diffuse and weaken the overtones.

> *As we practice toning vowel sounds, the overtones begin to emerge in all their playful and harmonic glory.*

The vowels, in a sense, could be compared with the human body: That energy that vibrates and gives life to the body—though hidden and unseen—is called the soul. Similarly, the overtones within the vowels are the hidden vibrations that give the sound its energy and resonance. As we practice toning vowel sounds, the overtones begin to emerge in all their playful and harmonic glory.

Making Vowels and Overtones

In his book, *The Roar of Silence*, author and teacher Don Campbell writes:

> The making of vowel and overtone sounds for three to five minutes brings a sense of well-being and balance to the body. When this is done with no stress or tension in

the jaw, skin temperature generally rises and the mind calms. As the specific epicenters of sound and pitch are studied and determined for each individual, it will become possible to stimulate the body internally through toning.

Olivea Dewhurst-Maddock says in *The Book of Sound Therapy*:

> Your mouth, throat, the sinuses, windpipe, and the lungs are resonant spaces that all contribute to the shaping of vowel sounds, initiated by the pressure of your breath in your larynx.... Remember that harmonics are generated by elegant proportional relationships. In singing overtones, you are recovering and demonstrating these proportions in your own resonant spaces.

18 Exercises for Creating Harmonics and Overtones
1. Vowel Sounds ("AY-EE-AH-OH-OO-UH")

Primary Resonators: Throat, and oral and nasal cavities.

Articulators: Mouth, jaw, lips, and tongue.

Pitch/Range: Total available.

Each vowel sound has its own cluster of naturally occurring overtones associated with it (just as each musical note does, as exhibited in the Overtone Spiral diagram in Chapter 11). This phenomenon is the basis for overtoning. So the best place to start experimenting with vocal harmonics and overtoning is with the vowel sounds—specifically, the Toning Vowels (discussed in Chapter 7).

Exercise:

Begin by selecting any vowel sound ("AH," for example), and tone it in your normal vocal range while elongating and sustaining it for as long as comfortable. Be sure you start with a deep diaphragmatic breath.

Next, experiment with slightly changing the shape of your mouth, the placement of your tongue, and the position of your jaw, as you sound the vowel, while keeping them fully relaxed. Don't concern yourself with proper intonation or sonic aesthetics. Just experiment and have fun.

See if you can hear the overtones emerging from your voice. If not, try changing to a lower or higher pitch and keep exploring the sounds creatively. Then select a second vowel and add it to the first one ("AH-OH," for example). Continue toning in the same manner, slowly transitioning between the two vowels. One of the most important factors and secrets to creating overtones is to slowly shift your voice from vowel to vowel, and sound to sound. The harmonics resonate most within and between the vowel sounds.

By now you should be hearing some interesting sounds, as the overtones may seem to be coming in and out. Perhaps the most effective technique for manifesting overtones is keeping the fundamental tone in the throat while using the lips, oral chamber, and nasal passages to resonate the harmonics. You could call this sound the "fundamental drone."

> *The harmonics resonate most within and between the vowel sounds.*

Always allow your mouth and jaw to be relaxed while toning, and remember to keep your hands in place (cupped behind your ear and in front of your mouth) to maximize your ability to hear all the overtones. The more you practice different vowel combinations, the more easily you will be able to create and distinguish various harmonics. Continue adding vowels, one at a time, until you are comfortable sustaining all the Toning Vowels in one breath without rushing the transitions.

2. Soft Consonants ("C, F, H, J, L, M, N, R, S, V, W, Y, Z")

Primary Resonators: Throat, and oral and nasal cavities.

Articulators: Mouth, teeth, lips, and tongue.

Pitch/Range: Total available.

This exercise involves using consonants to create overtones, specifically, the "soft" consonants. The "hard" consonants (for example, K or T) are not useful sounds when overtoning because they block and retard both the flow of breath and the sound vibration. Try releasing resonant sound with these consonants and you'll see what I mean.

The soft consonant sounds, however, are much better suited for creating overtones, as they can be resonated and sustained by the breath. When elongated and combined with one or more vowels, the soft consonants contribute greatly to the textured sounds of vocal overtoning.

Exercise:

Explore the soft consonant sounds in the same manner as the vowel sounds in the previous exercise. Begin with the "R" sound, as it is the best consonant for bringing out the harmonics in the voice. By adjusting your tongue and the shape of your mouth, slowly shift your voice between a very soft "R" (as in New Yawk), and a very hard "R," which causes the lips to be partially puckered and drawn.

In your normal vocal range, gently move your tongue forward and backward while toning this sound. You should begin hearing some fascinating overtones emerging from your voice.

Now, add the "N" consonant to the "R," and experiment with those sounds in the same way. Slowly shift back and forth between the "R" and "N" sounds and listen for the overtones. Notice the movement of your tongue as it moves up to the palate during the "N" sound, causing vibrations and overtones to be generated in the sinus cavities. (The sounds resonated by the nasal cavities are very important in most overtone exercises and integral to overtoning.) Notice, too, how, as the tongue comes down from the palate during the "R" sound, the overtones expand into the oral cavity and may be further manipulated by the mouth.

Experiment with different combinations of other soft consonants. Add vowel sounds to them and observe how the sound opens further to evoke more and more overtones. Be patient, and you will be rewarded with the unique joy of hearing yourself create remarkable multiphonic sounds with your voice. Slow and steady wins the grace.

Shortcuts

Certain combinations of sounds, along with their placements and articulation, can maximize your efforts in producing a wide array of overtones. These combinations will also assist you in creating the optimal vibrational energy patterns for healing and transformation to occur.

When learned and practiced sufficiently, the following exercises—combined with the vowel and soft consonant techniques described previously—will greatly enhance your ability to create overtones.

3. YOU ("YY-OOO" or "EE-OOO")

Primary Resonators: Oral and throat cavities.

Articulators: Lips and tongue.

Pitch/Range: Low to middle voice.

Exercise:

Shape your lips as if to whistle or make an "OO" sound. Take a deep diaphragmatic breath and exhale, while toning and sustaining a "Y" or "E" sound. Slowly shift to an "OO" sound as you continue to sustain your out-breath and tone. Use your tongue to articulate the creation of overtones by pulling it slowly backward from the front of your mouth ("EE") to the back of your mouth ("OO"). Midway through your exhalation, slowly move your tongue forward and backward again. Practice coordinating the sounding with your breathing until you can do two complete cycles of "YY-OOO" in one breath.

Allow your sound to resonate from the back of the throat cavity (pharynx) to the front of the oral cavity (mouth). Adjust your pitch, up or down, to accommodate the best production of overtones.

4. WOW ("WW-OWW" or "WWAH-OH-OOO")

Primary Resonators: Oral and throat cavities.

Articulators: Mouth and lips.

Pitch/Range: Low to middle voice.

Exercise:

While shaping the lips as if to whistle or make an "OO" sound, hold a drone sound in the pharynx (back of the throat). After inhaling, gradually and slowly open the lips and mouth fully while exhaling and making an "OW" sound. Midway through the exhalation, begin returning to the same oral position you began with. Complete this whole process in one breath and repeat until you hear resonant overtones. After you feel proficient with your technique, practice completing the exercise in two or three breaths.

Want more? Well, here it is:

5. MORE ("MMM-ORRR" or "MMM-AW-RR")

Variations: "MMMAHRRR," "MMMEERRR," "MMMOOORRR"

Primary Resonators: Lips and oral cavity.

Articulators: Lips and mouth.

Pitch/Range: Low to middle voice.

Exercise:

Focus your attention on your lips, allowing them to fully relax. Gently vibrate them by humming softly. Use a finger to softly touch your lips until you are fully vibrating them. Very slightly open your lips while humming until you feel a "buzzy" little vibration. You achieve this by constricting the outflow of breath through the mouth and lips. The rule of thumb is this: Too much air escaping loses the "MM" sound; lips closed send the sound and breath through the nose. Find a middle ground.

After you've learned this technique, continue by opening the lips and shaping them into in "AW" sound while bringing the resonance into the oral cavity. Slowly shift your intonation from the "AW" to an "RR" sound, and gradually sharpen the "RR" by slightly moving your tongue up while pulling your lips back. This will bring out some wonderful overtones. Make the "MMMORRR" sound in this way for one complete breath and repeat until proficient. Then try experimenting by substituting different vowel sounds.

6. NEAR ("NNNEEERRR")
Variation: NEARER ("NNEERR-URRR")

Primary Resonators: Oral and nasal cavities.

Articulators: Mouth and tongue.

Pitch/Range: Middle voice.

Exercise:

Place the tongue against your palate (roof of the mouth) while toning the "NN" sound. This helps access the overtones available by resonating the nasal passages, and by bringing the sound upward and forward from the mouth and throat cavities. Feel the sound vibrations in your nose and nasal cavities as you proceed through the rest of the sounding.

Slowly lower your tongue and allow the "EAR" or "EER" sound to resonate. Continue holding the "RR" for a few seconds, and then slowly return to the "NN" and repeat. Upon successfully producing overtones with this technique, add an "URR" to the end of "NEAR," and listen for more. Practice repeating this two to three times in one breath.

7. NURRY ("NNNURR-REEE")

Primary Resonators: Oral and nasal cavities.

Articulators: Mouth and tongue.

Pitch/Range: Middle to upper voice.

Exercise:

Similar to the previous exercise. Follow the same general guidelines, except that you will hear overtones move up in pitch rather than down as you move into the "EE" sound. The "NN" consonant and the "EE" vowel sounds are the most effective tones for resonating the nasal cavities and accessing the upper chakras.

Adjust your pitch according to where the overtones sound the strongest. You needn't use excessive volume; merely shift slowly through the two syllables ("NUR-REE"). Repeat until proficient. Have fun.

8. NAY-NEE ("NNAAYE-NNEEE")

Sound placement: Oral and nasal cavities.

Articulators: Nose, mouth, and tongue.

Pitch/range: Middle to upper voice.

Exercise:

Similar to the previous exercise in placement, except that the sound resonates less in the oral cavity and predominantly in the nasal cavities. To best access this somewhat unappealing sound, don't concern yourself with vocal aesthetics or tonal beauty. For the best results, think "whiny" and "complainy." Or, see if you can recall teasing or being teased as a child with "na-na-na-na-na-na." That's the vibe!

It's also beneficial to sort of scrunch up your nose and face while doing this exercise. You may also want to keep a tissue handy, as the sounds—when done properly—may vibrate and tickle your nasal passages. Practice repeating these tones several times during each breath until you hear nasal overtones being created (or until you've healed your childhood!).

9. The Bee's Breath ("NN-NN-NN-NN")

Primary Resonators: Nasal and throat cavities.

Articulators: Tongue.

Pitch/Range: Middle to upper voice.

Exercise:

As you tone a constant "NN" sound, move the middle of your tongue up and down from the roof of your mouth while keeping the tip pressed firmly against the back of your upper teeth. The mouth and lips should be closed. The tones will resonate back and forth between the nasal and throat cavities, coming out through the nostrils, not the mouth. The buzzing sound that emerges is somewhat similar to a buzzing bee.

10. HURRY ("HURRR-REEE")

Variation: HEARY ("HEER-REEE")

Primary Resonators: Oral and nasal cavities.

Articulators: Mouth and tongue.

Pitch/Range: Middle to upper voice.

Exercise:

The same basic technique as "NURRY," though it is less nasal without the "NN" sound.

11. RINGING-ING ("RRREEENNG-ING," "RRRING-ING-ING-ING")

Primary Resonators: Throat, and nasal and oral cavities.

Articulators: Glottis and tongue.

Pitch/Range: Middle voice.

Exercise:

Upon toning "RRREE," close the throat or glottis and sustain the "NNG" sound. This creates a drone. Now open the throat momentarily to emit an "EE" through the mouth and then immediately close the throat again, continuing with the "ING." Then return to the "RRREEENNG." As you learn the technique of glottis constriction or "glottal-popping" (the abrupt opening and closing of the glottis or throat passage), you may vary the patterns and emphasis of the sounds and syllables—"RRREEENNG-RRREEENNG-ING-ING" or "RRRING-ING-ING-ING-RING-ING-ING."

12. NGONG ("NNG-AW-NNG" or "NNG-AH-NNG")

Variations: ("NNG-EH-NNG," "NNG-AY-NNG," "NNG-UH-NNG")

Primary Resonators: Throat, and nasal and oral cavities.

Articulators: Glottis, mouth, and tongue.

Pitch/Range: Middle voice.

Exercise:

The same basic throat technique as the previous exercise, except that you begin with the "NNG" in addition to ending with it. Once you perfect the technique with the "ONG" (rhymes with *song*) in the middle (open glottis), you may vary the vowel sounds in this "glottis sandwich." Don't forget to have fun!

13. OO-EE ("OOOO-EEEE-OOOO-EEEE")

Primary Resonators: Oral and nasal cavities.

Articulators: Lips and tongue.

Pitch/Range: Upper voice (falsetto, or head voice).

Exercise:

This tone is similar to an inversion of the first exercise ("YY-OOO"), or the female-energy to its male-energy counterpart. Whereas the "YOU" sound begins with a low "EE" and then "OO," this exercise begins with a high "OO" and then "EE." These high tones can create extraordinary angelic sounds. Find a comfortable pitch near the top of your vocal range, and slowly shift back and forth between the "OO" and "EE" sounds.

As with the previous exercises, the overtones are best evoked by holding the sound forward, so that it may resonate in the nasal cavities. And the other important key with all overtoning is to control the slow transitions between the different vowels (and consonants) to create resonant and precise harmonics.

14. ZZSHSSZZ ("ZZ-SHH-SSS-ZZZ")

Primary Resonators: Mouth and throat cavity.

Articulators: Lips, teeth, and breath.

Pitch/Range: Low to middle voice.

Exercise:

There are two significant parts to this practice. The first is to create a drone in the throat cavity. Remember the fundamental drone? One way to achieve a drone is by closing the throat passage and humming with your mouth open. This creates a constant tone that is emitted through the nasal passages, allowing you to create additional tones (overtones) with and through the mouth.

The second step (while droning at the same time) is to lightly clench your teeth together and open the throat, allowing the breath to push through your teeth and lips, creating a wind-like sound. This second sound may be further enhanced by puckering and pursing your lips as you manipulate the two sounds. Explore different combinations of "Z," "S," and "SH" for the best results. A third tone may also be created by finding a whistle while changing your lip positions.

15. Pulsing Technique

Primary Resonators: Oral, throat, and nasal cavities.

Articulators: Glottis, tongue, and lips.

Pitch/Range: Low to middle voice.

Exercise:

The pulsing technique is very effective for concentrating vibrational energy and accelerating its movement with toning. Pulsing is basically a variation on the articulation process of overtoning. It is a method for manipulating certain tones by either speeding them up or slowing them down with a rhythmic pulse.

You might compare this to holding your thumb over the end of a garden hose and manipulating the flow of water. By covering half of the opening, or by pulsing it open and closed, you may better concentrate the outpour. It is similar with toning.

Some sounds lend themselves more easily to the practice of pulsing. For example, the sounds "YOU" and "WOW" are excellent choices to pulse. You may effectively transform and pulse the "YOU" sound by rapidly moving your tongue forward and backward while toning "YOU"— that is, "YOU-YOU-YOU-YOU-YOU-YOU." By simultaneously making slight shifts in the speed and position of your tongue, you will create some intriguing variations. As with other "low" sounds, you may create additional tones by finding the whistle during this technique.

I use this sound, with its rhythmic overtones, quite frequently when doing vibrational alignments and other sound healing work.

The "WOW" sound can be easily pulsed by using the lips and mouth to rhythmically open and close the oral opening in various degrees. Try gradually speeding up and slowing down the rhythmic pulsing as you tone, "WOW-WOW-WOW-WOW-WOW-WOW." Listen for the constant drone at the back of the throat and the echoing pulses in the oral chamber. Having fun yet?

This one got me thrown out of class in the sixth-grade!

Other sounds that pulse well include the throat tones of "RING" and "NGONG" (using the glottis for pulsing, rather than the tongue or lips), and the next two exercise tones.

16. MURMUR-ME-ME ("MMURR-MMURR-ME-ME")

Primary Resonators: Mouth and nasal cavities.

Articulators: Lips and tongue.

Pitch/Range: Low to middle voice.

Exercise:

Generally follow the description for the "MORE" exercise, except after several "MUR" sounds, tone several "ME" sounds. The "MUR" resonates primarily in the oral cavity, and the "ME" in the nasal cavity, elevating the energy to a higher overtone and chakra. Upon becoming proficient in evoking overtones by slowly toning these sounds, try pulsing them—shifting between the "MUR" and "ME" tones at different pulsing speeds. This creates a sound similar to a Jew's harp.

17. NEE-YUM ("NNEEE-YUMM-NNEEE-YUMM")

Primary Resonators: Nasal, throat, and oral cavities.

Articulators: Tongue, lips, and mouth.

Pitch/Range: Low to middle voice.

Exercise:

Be careful not to rush through any of the consonant/vowel connections, particularly when shifting from the "MM" to the "NN," which feels somewhat unnatural. By "squeezing" into the "NN" by pushing the tongue up, you will get a nice nasal harmonic. Upon feeling comfortable (and harmonic) with this technique, begin pulsing it faster and faster. Play with the different speeds, and you'll notice that it sounds quite different when pulsed, somewhat similar to how an alien might sound!?!

18. Potpourri/Combinations of Tones

Primary Resonators: All areas.

Articulators: All.

Pitch/Range: Total available.

Exercise:

The "combination exercise" offers you the opportunity to combine various tones and techniques. Follow all the appropriate and previously discussed techniques for overtoning: droning, slow transitions, projecting the sound forward, relaxing resonators and articulators, and focusing attention and breathing. But this is the practice that allows you to bend the rules—and even throw out the rule book, if you like.

For example, you may string tones together, or try the lower ones in a higher pitch, or the higher ones in a lower pitch. Do them backward, or inside out! This is an opportunity to free yourself up with sound. Be intuitive and creative by adding any sound that comes to you. And take as long as you like. Push the envelope with your spirit!

This is also an excellent exercise for practicing in a group as a closed-eye, toning meditation. Always, however, complete the process with an extended silence. I have witnessed and experienced profound healing from this overtoning practice.

≈

Let's review: To enhance your overtoning expertise and achieve the most benefit from the exercises, the following tips may be useful:

≈ Listen regularly to live or recorded vocal overtones.

≈ Approach the overtoning process with a relaxed, open, and patient attitude.

≈ Close your eyes and breathe deeply and diaphragmatically. (Follow the steps outlined in Chapter 7.)

≈ Set aside your personality or ego-self by silently reciting a prayer or invocation of Spirit.

≈ Place your hands in the resonant listening position (one cupping the ear, the other in front of the mouth as a sounding board).

≈ Begin making soft vowel sounds in a comfortable pitch or vocal range.

≈ Allow the feeling of the sounds to guide your voice through subtle changes in pitch, volume, and vowels.

≈ Listen for emerging overtones in your voice as you slowly shift through these changes.

≈ Creatively explore various combinations of vowels and soft consonant sounds.

≈ Practice all of the overtoning exercises previously described in this chapter.

≈ If you have difficulty initially hearing the overtones, adjust your pitch or "sounding-board hand." If this doesn't help, simply relax your vocal apparatus and slow down your sound transitions.

≈ Upon learning the vocal exercises, record your voice and listen to yourself regularly until you're satisfied with the improvements.

≈ Allow yourself to visualize any images, shapes, lights, or colors that appear within. Engage all your senses.

≈ Being fully present in the moment, allow yourself to feel at one with the sound of the overtones you hear.

≈ Allow any regeneration, healing, or transformation to manifest.

≈ Upon feeling complete with the sounding experience, listen in silent meditation to the ever-present sound within you. Try to catch the infinite overtones of the Sacred Sound Current.

≈ Offer grateful appreciation to your Divine Spirit Source before opening your eyes.

> *Listen in silent meditation to the ever-present sound within you.*

Throughout this and the previous chapter we have explored the extraordinary process and potentials of vocal overtoning. We've examined some principles and perspectives ranging from the musical to the mathematical, the physical to the metaphysical, and the scientific to the spiritual. We've discussed the value of listening to and making these magical sounds, and we've also learned specific exercises designed to create resonant frequencies for vibrational healing purposes.

When understood and used as a tool for self-transformation, harmonics and overtones can teach us much about ourselves, the Universe, and our relationship to it.

Summary of the Exercises
Shortcuts and Secrets to Overtoning
1. Vowel Sounds ("AY-EE-AH-OH-OO-UH")
2. Soft Consonants ("C, F, H, J, L, M, N, R, S, V, W, Y, Z")
3. YOU ("YY-OOO"/"EE-OOO")
4. WOW ("WW-OWW"/"WWAH-OH-OOO")
5. MORE ("MMM-ORRR"/"MMM-AW-RRR")
6. NEAR/NEARER ("NNNEEERRR"/"NNEER-URRR")
7. NURRY ("NNNURR-REEE")
8. NAYNEE ("NNAAYE-NNEEE")

9. The Bee's Breath ("NN-NN-NN-NN")
10. HURRY/HEARY ("HURRR-REEE"/"HEERR-REEE")
11. RINGING ("RRREEENNG-ING"/"RRRING-ING-ING-ING")
12. NGONG ("NNG-ONNG"/"NNG-AWNNG")
13. OO-EE ("OOO)-EEEE-OOOO-EEEE")
14. ZZSHSSZZ ("ZZ-SHH-SSS-ZZZ")
15. Pulsing Technique
16. MURMUR-ME-ME ("MMURR-MMURR-ME-ME")
17. NEE-YUM ("NNEEE-YUMM-NNEEE-YUMM")
18. Potpourri/Combinations of Tones

In the final section of this chapter, we will briefly discuss the mysterious overtoning technique and ancient art known as *throat-singing*.

Throat-Singing

When practiced in a musical context, the process of overtoning is often referred to as overtone singing, harmonic chanting, throat-singing, or overtone chanting. These remarkable vocalizations stem from sacred sounding practices used for thousands of years by ancient cultures throughout the world, such as those in Tibet, Mongolia, India, China, Japan, Europe, Central Africa, and the Andes of South America.

Some of the more notable of these vocal styles come from Tibetan monks, Mongolians, and Tuvans, who still practice a throat-singing technique that evokes two to four tones simultaneously.

Though no one knows for certain when or where these practices originated, it may have been in Tuva, a tiny country inside the ring of mountains where Siberia meets Outer Mongolia. This is a very cold but beautiful land of shepherds and shamans. For centuries the Tuvans have been known for practicing "koomei" or "hoomei," an extraordinary form of throat-singing. Some believe that the monks of Tibet may have learned this vocal style in Tuva long ago while traveling through that region to share the teachings of Buddha. They may have eventually incorporated it into their devotional practices, which have become an integral part of Tibetan culture.

Others believe that these extraordinary vocal sounds were developed in ancient Egypt. Still others feel the technique may have been "alien" in its source, and taught to the ancients by some extraterrestrial race, such as the Hathors. Perhaps it simply comes from within at the appropriate time for activation, or with a developed level of consciousness.

Where these tones and techniques came from, we may never surely know. But those interested in creating overtones with throat-singing may find hoomei a most elaborate, fascinating, and useful vocal technique. I recommend, however, using extreme caution before attempting any throat-singing style, as improper execution may cause damage to the vocal cords and the voice.

The Tuvan Styles

Tuvan folklore says throat-singing came from a polyphonic echo. It's a way of saying that the key to learning throat-singing is to hear the overtones first. This seems to be consistent with the overtoning techniques discussed earlier.

The Tuvans actually consider hoomei as not one, but three distinct and different basic styles of throat-singing. They sometimes combine these fundamental techniques and embellish them. With no disrespect intended, I've included some Westernized approaches to better facilitate the unique practice of Tuvan throat-singing for the adventurous.

Throat-Singing Exercises

The primary three styles are performed as follows:

1. **Hoomei ("HER-MAY").** This style (which also refers to Tuvan throat-singing in general) is created by tightening the throat and imitating the deep voice of the late Wolfman Jack or the late bluesman Howlin' Wolf, while sounding "OO-UH-OO-UH" in a rhythm. For the melody, move your tongue forward and backward. With your mouth shaped for an "OO" sound, three to four notes may be created with this technique of throat-singing.

2. **Sygyt ("SUH-GUT").** This style is created by tightening the throat and imitating the voice of Kermit the Frog, while sounding "UR-EE-UR-EE." With your mouth shaped to say "UR," two to three notes may be created with this technique.

3. **Kargyraa ("KAR-GUH-RAH").** This style is created by tightening the throat and imitating Popeye the Sailor, while sounding a low "UH-OH-OO-AH" and other vowels. Find a

deep pitch with your voice, and you'll soon begin emitting some extraordinary "undertones" and "sub-harmonics"—usually an octave below the fundamental tone. Beginning in your normal speaking voice, as you tighten the throat, three to four notes may be created with this technique.

Adding various embellishments to these primary techniques can also create an amazing array of harmonics. Some of these include: tongue, lips and glottis trills, vibrato effects, pulsing, pitch shifts, and the combining of these styles.

There is also the subtle and rarely heard Tuvan style of "dymzbuktaar" ("DOOM-JOOK-TAR"). This technique involves ***throat-humming***, in which overtones are produced in all the basic styles, but with the mouth closed and the sounds emitted primarily through the nostrils.

≈

Sounding Your Soul

In 1994, after being awarded the title "National Artist of Russia," world champion Tuvan throat-singer Kongar-ool Ondar said in an interview, "When you perform hoomei, you must be in a good state of mind. Your spirit must be in a very uplifted mood; your soul, your inner spiritual voice, must be strong. It's not simply singing. When you perform hoomei, that which you want to express must truly come from within, from your soul." This is truly sounding your soul.

These words of wisdom speak to the most important aspect of any type of overtoning: one's attitude and intention. With practice you can learn technique, but it takes spiritual passion, devotion, an open heart, clear intent, and humility to achieve true mastery of overtoning.

> *Become the vehicle through which sacred sound may manifest.*

Regardless of the cultures or techniques behind the style of overtoning, the spiritually aware practitioners know the necessity of becoming one with sacred sound. Whether it's Tuvan throat-singing, Mongolian overtone chanting, the "One Voice Chord" of the Tibetan monks, or the various sacred sounds of the Aborigines, Africans, Eskimos, Mayans, Native American shamans, and others, the true masters of these vocal practices emphasize one eternal truth: It is not we who "make" the sound. Rather, we simply become the vehicle through which sacred sound may manifest.

By imbibing this attitude with your vocal practices, you too will experience the phenomenon of *Overtoning: A Sonic Harmonic Tonic.*

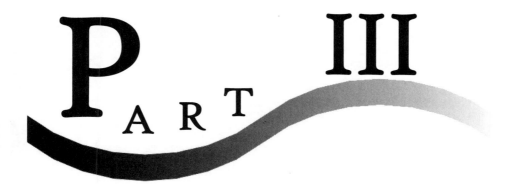

Personal and Interpersonal Frequencies

Every organ and body system vibrates at a specific rate of frequency, contributing to a comprehensive personal matrix of vibrations that determines one's signature frequency.

(((((13)))))

Discovering Your Signature Frequency

Life cannot be destroyed—it merely changes form or
expands in its own vibrational pattern.

—Wayne Perry

All matter consists of vibrating, pulsing energy fields. A rock, tree, vegetable, mineral, human body cell, or atomic or sub-atomic particle—each has its own distinctive frequency wave pattern. This pattern of frequency determines the character and function of any form of matter and identifies its *signature frequency*.

In *Radionics, Radiesthesia and Physics,* researcher Dr. William Tiller stated, "...each individual, organism or material, radiates and absorbs energy via a unique wave field which exhibits certain geometrical frequency and radiation-type characteristics. This is an extended force field that exists around all forms of matter whether animate or inanimate."

Of particular significance may be how these wave fields and frequency patterns resonate and influence the human body.

Sound Waves and Sonic Fields

The whole of your body is the culmination and expression of these frequency wave patterns that collectively represent your personal vibration and signature frequency. This vibrational signature is not merely one note or tone, any more than your written signature is one letter, or your fingerprint consists of one line. Akin to a "sonic fingerprint," this signature frequency is unique to each individual, and no two people are alike. Your every body system, organ, thought, feeling, and emotion has its own frequency contributing to the total vibrational essence that is you.

> *Akin to a "sonic fingerprint," this signature frequency is unique to each individual, and no two people are alike.*

For a number of years there has been increasing interest in the relationship between sound and the human body. Sir Peter Guy Manners, M.D., an English osteopath and Cymatic sound therapist, says in his book, *Cymatic Therapy*: "Experimentation indicates that human beings, as all objects, are radiating sound waves, therefore their fields are sonic fields. Each individual has his own different pattern, or collection of tones, just as each individual has a unique shape."

Cymatics

Dr. Manners's mentor and founder of Cymatics (named after the Greek word for "wave"), was the late Swiss scientist and physician, Dr. Hans Jenny. In the 1960s, Dr. Jenny (now well known and regarded by sound researchers) postulated that each human cell has its own frequency, and that the frequency of every human organ may be a harmonic of its component cells. This presents us with the viable possibility that these signature frequencies may solve the mystery of how sound can be used to heal on the genetic and cellular levels.

Jenny reached this intriguing conclusion based on a series of remarkable experiments that he conducted, one of which expanded upon the original work of Ernst Chladni, an 18th-century German physicist who demonstrated that sound waves could move and shape matter. By simply sprinkling grains of sand on metal plates and then vibrating them with a violin bow, Chladni showed the sand rearranging into symmetrical shapes and geometric patterns.

Sound Pictures

In his Cymatics research, Jenny used crystal oscillators and a device he invented called a tonoscope, which produced pictures of sounds created by the human voice. These pictures showed strikingly complex forms created out of materials such as iron filings, sand, powders, plastics, gels, milk, and mercury. The forms and designs created mimicked forms expressed in nature, such as spirals, snowflakes, starfish, flowers, insects, mandalas, and human organs.

> *Sound has the ability to create form.*

As the pitches of the imposed sounds were modulated, the patterns and designs became infinitely more detailed and complex depending on the frequency, amplitude, and type of material used. This has given us positive proof that sound has the ability to create form.

If these types of changes in form and structure can take place with simple inanimate matter such as sand and gels, what can occur on the molecular level if we introduce similar sounds and frequencies to the various systems of the human body? Can we affect the body's DNA? Can we possibly "tune out" disease?

Vibratory Structures

Rupert Sheldrake, biologist and author of *A New Science of Life and The Rebirth of Nature,* says:

> The forms in nature are not due to vibrations being imposed from outside on passive particles; they are owing to the whole vibratory structure of activity which makes up the particle itself. Atoms are vibratory structures of activity. Molecules are vibratory structures of activity. Now, in the case of a living organism, the whole thing is a complex, rhythmic, structural pattern of activity.... there is a nested hierarchy of vibrations within vibrations, at every level there is a structure of activity which is vibratory or rhythmic.

Many in the realm of science and physics now share this view. In *The Tao of Physics*, author Fritjof Capra says, "Rhythmic patterns appear throughout the universe, from the very small to the very large. Atoms are patterns of probability waves, molecules are vibrating structures, and living organisms manifest multiple, interdependent patterns of fluctuations."

So, we live in and are part of a vast, universal, complex, vibratory, structural pattern of activity. And in its individuated form—the human body—each of us has our own unique vibrational pattern or signature frequency.

> *When disease overwhelms a body system, those resonant frequencies become dissonant or out of balance.*

A Cellular Symphony

From a different perspective, we could view the body as an incredible orchestra of bio-chemical frequencies, sounds, and rhythms. Billions of living cells in constant motion, supporting and contributing to the whole that is the physical body. The cells are constantly producing countless frequencies that form a vastly complex symphony of interdependent vibrational systems.

Similar to the way a horn or string section can disrupt the harmony of an orchestra if they were to play out of tune, a stressed organ or body system can disrupt the health and harmony of the body. Each organ and system has its own resonating frequency or natural rate of vibration. When disease overwhelms a body system, those resonant frequencies become dissonant or out of balance. The frequencies and vibrations thus become too weak or strong and must be brought into balance to effect "sound health."

Soul Composer

We might creatively expand this analogy in a number of directions. One perspective could include adding a choir section to symbolize the emotions. We could view the orchestra conductor as the brain, perhaps seeing the composer of the symphony as the soul or spirit. Resonate your imagination! The point is: How can we create balance, resonance, and harmony in body, mind, and spirit?

Each and every part of the body speaks volumes, sings verses, emanates light, and emits frequencies that express the whole.

From a spiritual standpoint, the total Universe or Infinite Consciousness may be seen as the macrocosm, and the soul possessed of a human body as the microcosm. This may explain biblical assertions stating: "You are created in the image of God," and "The Kingdom of Heaven lies within you."

The Whole Within the Part

According to the science of holography, the "whole" is contained within the "part," and every body system is connected to and affected by another. This is consistent with vibrational healing principles indicating that every organ and body system vibrates at a specific rate of frequency, contributing to a comprehensive personal matrix of vibrations that determines one's signature frequency.

Vibrational healing practices emphasize healing the whole by harmonizing body, mind, and spirit. This is one of the fundamental precepts and goals of true holistic health. The most effective healing practices address the source or cause of diseases and imbalances, rather than the effect.

For example, in traditional Chinese medicine, being aware that we can see the whole in the parts, an acupuncturist can often determine the whole picture of the body from taking the pulse and looking at the tongue. Many alternative and integrative modalities can determine imbalances from looking at the eyes, hair, face, or shape of the skull, or by lines in the hands or feet. Even practices such as psychotherapy, hypnotherapy, and massage therapy now consider the interconnectedness and holistic relationships between physical and emotional imbalances.

Know and Tell

We too can know and heal ourselves. Each and every part of the body speaks volumes, sings verses, emanates light, and emits frequencies that express the whole. We can better understand and harmonize these parts if we simply take the time to listen to the most "telling" part of our signature frequency. But which is the most telling part? And how do we hear it?

Well, which part of ourselves do we use when we tell something? We use the voice. The voice is both the most auditory and vibrational expression of who we are. This vocal part of us has its own frequency, as everything does, but what is unique about the human voice is that it is an identifiable, sonic, energetic projection of the individuated body, mind, and soul. The voice, therefore, is infused with more consciousness than any other sound, imbuing it with incredible transformational characteristics. It also reveals the secrets of our signature frequency.

> *The voice is infused with more consciousness than any other sound, imbuing it with incredible transformational characteristics.*

Referring again to our analogy of the macrocosm and the microcosm, we could view the human body—or its conductor, the brain— as the macrocosm, and the voice as the microcosm. If one knows how to listen to and interpret the voice, one can discover that it reflects the frequency patterns within the brain and body. Again, the whole contained within the part.

Sound therapy research and studies since the 1980s have repeatedly pointed to the human voice as the key component in healing with sound. Why? When understood and used properly, the human voice is an ideal diagnostic and therapeutic tool.

Missing Tones

According to sound pioneer Sharry Edwards, as stated on my Los Angeles radio show in 1992, "Each individual has a distinctive signature sound that is evident in their speaking voice, and vocally missing tones correspond to the individual's physiological and psychological status."

Edwards, founder of Bio-Acoustics and Signature Sound Technologies, was an early researcher in developing diagnostic and therapeutic sound work based upon frequency patterns in the voice. Edwards went on to say, "We have found that providing the missing frequencies provides the body with the means to repair itself."

When I asked her what kinds of results she saw after restoring these missing tones, Edwards replied, "If a person's tone can be determined and a sound formation constructed using their individual tones as a base, then that sound can be set in their environment. The results that we have been experiencing are that the disease of that person is abated." She went on to relate examples of case histories with which she had been involved.

Edwards was one of the first to use voice analysis as a means for determining missing frequencies. Since that time we have seen an explosion of interest in the role the voice plays in sound and vibrational healing.

Voice Analysis

The distinctive characteristics of the voice may be observed simply by using a microphone and musical instrument tuner, or with a computer program designed to reveal vocal frequency patterns. In this manner, a sound therapist or practitioner may view, chart, and interpret energy imbalances in the voice during a voice analysis and assessment.

A wide variety of questions are asked and topics are covered during a voice analysis and assessment. This is necessary for the subject's voice to reflect the full spectrum of brain wave patterns contained in the pitch of the subject's speaking voice.

For example, if you're talking about visual issues or thoughts, such as forms, shapes, or colors, the frequencies indicated in your voice will be somewhat different than if you were talking about what you did last week. Or if you express a strong belief or feeling about something, the frequency patterns in your voice will be different from those when you are discussing, let's say, the location of your job.

These differences in frequencies occur in the various notes, pitches, and octaves of the voice, and are subtle to the ear. Most people would not hear the differences, but a microphone and sound equipment will easily pick up and indicate distinctive changes in the vocal patterns. When enough information is gathered by a sound practitioner, your unique frequency patterns can be charted and interpreted.

This personalized chart, or *voiceprint*, represents a "snapshot" of the voice at any given time. It's also a visual reflection of one's signature frequency.

Imbalances reflect possible health issues and are revealed as either "deficiencies" or "excesses" of frequency in one's speaking voice. Once it is determined which frequencies are deficient and need regeneration, and which are in excess and need release, vibrational balance may then be restored. This balance supports the overall resonance of the body, thus allowing it to heal itself.

After this balance is achieved it may be advisable, particularly during times of increased stress, to periodically reassess the voice to monitor and maintain wellness. Also, it helps to tune any out-of-tune frequencies for optimal resonance in the body-mind. In addition to the techniques given in Part II, we will explore in upcoming chapters a number of ways in which this may be achieved.

Name That Tone

Upon determining which frequencies are deficient and which are in excess, it may be useful to translate those frequencies into an understandable medium. The standard musical scale is a convenient and ready-made system for frequency identification. In other words, we can easily identify and name each frequency by using a musical note, such as C-sharp (C♯), G, or B-flat (B♭).

If you're not a musician or singer, you needn't be intimidated by musical notations. Although some sound therapies may rely on musical notes for easy reference, it is not necessary to be trained in music theory to understand or use sound healing principles. Sound therapy is generally not rooted in traditional music therapy, either. Music training is a benefit for some, but may get in the way for others.

Studies have indicated that certain frequencies/notes correspond to specific organs and body systems. For example, the vibratory frequency

As above...   So below...

CORRELATIVE HEALING CHART for SOUND THERAPY

© 1993 WAYNE PERRY/MUSIKARMA PRODUCTIONS

KEY	1	2	3	4	5	6	7	8	9	10	11	12
Musical Note/Key:	C	C#	D	Eb	E	F	F#	G	Ab	A	Bb	B
Sacred Sound:	Uh	Hu	Oo	Woh	Oh	Aw	Ah	Eh	Ay	Ee	mmm/om	nnn/silence
Color:	Red	Red/Orange	Orange	Yellow/Orange	Yellow	Yellow/Green	Green	Blue/Green	Blue	Indigo	Violet	Magenta
Physical Correlates for Treatment:	Gross circulation; Large/thick muscles; Hormones; Heart muscle; Sore muscles; Constipation; Colon; Anemia; Adrenals	Circulation of digestion; Tendons & ligaments; Sore muscles; Asthma; Colds; Constipation; Testes/ovaries; Reproduction	Digestion; Liver; Pancreas; Gallbladder; Spleen; Cramps; Blood sugar	Oxygenation of digestion; Respiration; Colitis; Ulcers; Lymph; Small intestine	Oxygenation; Lungs; Respiration; Nerves; Lymph; Ulcers; Stomach	Kidneys; Bladder; Reduces blood pressure; Insomnia; Thymus; Heart	Screening & filtering; Insomnia; Thymus imbalances; Heart; Allergies	Neuro-transmitters; Utilization of B vitamins; Bones; Back pain; Speech; Thyroid; Skin	Enzyme production; Thyroid; Speech; Laryngitis; Tonsilitis; Back pain; Allergies; Colds/sinus	Body's rebuilding; Toxins; Eyes & ears; Deafness; Stop bleeding; Insanity; Pituitary	Body regulation; Utilization of minerals; Eyes & ears; Deafness; Epilepsy; Nervous system	Subtle circulation; Body mechanics; Nerves/electrical body; Blood purification; Epilepsy
Emotional Correlates for Treatment:	Self power issues; Listlessness; Ability to self-direct; Survival issues; Repression; Dependence; Sexuality; Groundedness	Secretly hard on self; Sarcastic or bullying; Indulgences; Low energy; Fear; Groundedness; Boundaries; Attachment	Self-approval issues; Complainer; Sexuality issues; Low self esteem; Shyness; Fear; Addictions; Intimacy	Information brokers; Don't share real emotions lightly; Mental clarity; Stubbornness; Control issues; Trust Issues	Self-sabotage; Needs to be needed; Lack of willpower; Depression; Slow learning; Impractical	Procrastination; Lack of compassion; Trust issues; Authenticity; Intolerance; Lack of forgiveness	Will work on unimportant and leave important issues undone; Will turn off & vegetate; Inflexibility; Lack of responsiveness	Prioritizing physical issues; Depression; Communication issues; Creativity blockage; Dishonesty	Spreads self too thin; Sees self as not important; Sways from low self esteem to egotistical; Lack of spontaneity	Prioritizing non-physical issues; Creativity blockage; Trust issues; Lack of motivation; Apathy	Others more important; Gives too much; Tries too hard to please; Mental & nervous disorders; Indecision	Martyr; Think they deserve, but don't know how to accomplish without appearing selfish; Scattered attention
Self-healing Steps:	Researching	Recognizing	Risking	Revealing	Resonating	Resolving	Releasing	Reforming	Realizing	Reaping	Raising	Rejoicing
Astrological Correlates:	Aries	Taurus	Gemini	Cancer	Leo	Virgo	Libra	Scorpio	Sagittarius	Capricorn	Aquarius	Pisces
Energy Center/Chakra:	1ST CHAKRA Base/Root	2ND CHAKRA Sacral		3RD CHAKRA Solar Plexus		4TH CHAKRA Heart		5TH CHAKRA Throat		6TH CHAKRA Brow/"Third Eye"		7TH CHAKRA Crown
Gland:	Adrenals	Gonads/Ovaries		Digestive/Respiratory		Thymus		Thyroid		Pituitary/Pineal		Pineal Gland
Toning Sound:	UH (Low)	OOO		OH		AH		AY		EEE		EEE (High)
Element:	EARTH	WATER		FIRE		AIR		ETHER		ALL ELEMENTS		SOUND/LIGHT
Level of Consciousness:	PHYSICAL (SENSUAL)	EMOTIONAL (ASTRAL)		MENTAL (INTELLECTUAL)		CASUAL (LOWER CREATIVE)		CASUAL (HIGHER CREATIVE)		SPIRITUAL (INDIVIDUATED)		SPIRITUAL (ONE/WHOLE)

rates of calcium and magnesium have been reported to assist and accelerate the healing of broken bones. Other frequencies imposed upon the body have been reported to lower blood pressure, improve circulation and digestion, and reduce pain, stress, and depression, as well as effect wellness in a host of other physical, mental, and emotional areas.

In 1993, based on my own and pre-existing research, I published the "Correlative Healing Chart for Sound Therapy" (see page 142) to assist in a basic understanding of these frequencies/notes and some of their body correlations. Sound practitioners worldwide use it. Information regarding specific associations of toning sounds, colors, chakras, primordial elements, and levels of consciousness is included in this chart.

Though it contains an array of data from various resources, this chart is not intended to be totally comprehensive, but useful as a quick and easy reference guide. When using this chart, also factor in your own experience and intuition for optimal benefit.

Sound Correlations

Although correlating specific frequencies/notes may be useful, it is also vital to factor in one's signature frequency, as each individual's "sound prescription" is unique to them. For best results, we need to view the most appropriate sound therapy options from both perspectives: existing research and case histories, and the subjective, personal feedback and experiences of the individual.

These body-mind frequencies are not an exact science as of yet, and there is still some disagreement and discussion—as there should be— about some of their correlations. However, as time progresses and more experiences are reported and documented, great significance may be gained from this information for the further development of useful sound therapy practices and applications.

(((((14)))))

Subtle-Energy Alternatives

My heart, like a pendulum, swings back and forth between my mind's desires and my soul's purpose.

—Wayne Perry

There are a number of subtle-energy modalities that may assist us in better understanding our signature frequency and locating areas in need of "resonant attention." Some of these modalities include toning and meditation, light and color therapies, muscle testing, dowsing, and astrology.

As with voice analysis, many subtle-energy methodologies may require assistance from one trained in that particular modality. However, most of the methods mentioned here can be easily learned and used for enhanced vibrational awareness.

Let us look at these modalities in terms of their relationship to sound and frequency.

> *Toning and meditation are two of the most powerful tools you possess for enhancing intuition, healing, and transformation.*

Toning and Meditation

Can we use the voice to "tune in" to our signature frequencies, without help from a sound therapist? Of course, if that's our intention. There's more than one way to skin a— oops!—"spin a chat!" This book is dedicated to simple ways in which anyone can access these "secrets of the voice" through vocal toning and meditation.

Among its many uses, toning helps us to resonate our vibrational awareness. From this practice, we may better concentrate our attention and become more sensitive to the subtle energy of the body's natural resonance. This is the ideal foundation for accessing deeper states of awareness through meditation, which is simply a letting go of thoughts and emotions, and being fully present in the moment.

Signature Frequency/Self-Scan Exercise

One easy exercise you can do to access your signature frequency I call the Self Scan, and is executed as follows: Select any vowel sound you feel comfortable in toning, and ride the pitch of your voice from the low end of your range up to the highest note you can comfortably tone. This process is similar to the Siren Vowel Exercise described in Chapter 7. In this exercise, however, your intention is different, in that you needn't return back down in vocal pitch.

Begin the process by simply asking your inner or higher self for guidance in finding your best tone and pitch. After putting that out to the Universe, listen and feel the sound as your voice gradually rises in pitch. Imagine a sort of "sonic barometer," and notice when you begin to feel an energetic connection somewhere in your body. Hold that tone and pitch for a few minutes, until you feel an uplifting shift in the energy, or a release of any blocked energy. You'll know it when you feel it.

Trust yourself and the sound. Also, listen for any subtle harmonics in your voice. If you hear them, focus your attention on them and allow them to guide you. Vocally generated harmonics and overtones are some of the most powerful and regenerative sounds in the Universe. You'll be guided to the optimal vocal pitch and body locations for vibrational balance and frequency integration.

Be patient. With practice, this exercise will sensitize you to the sounds that are best for you to tone in support of your personal vibration and signature frequency. The toning process will also support and strengthen your intuitive faculties. Your left brain may not be immediately aware of what's going on vibrationally and intuitively. More important is getting your thoughts out of the way, so that you can feel and find the appropriate sound in the moment.

This practice is one form of sonic meditation. Rely on your inner guidance. Remember that toning and meditation are two of the most powerful tools you possess for enhancing intuition, healing, and transformation. No machine, instrument, or recording can do all that the human voice can do. No tone generator possesses intuition. No computer has a soul.

If initially you are not comfortable and confident identifying and toning your frequencies intuitively, you may rely on the information gained from a voice analysis to assist you (as discussed in the previous chapter). Use whatever diagnostic and scanning methods are available. With time and practice, you will feel more assured in trusting yourself and your sound.

≈

Light and Color

Color is simply a light frequency—visible radiant energy—of certain wavelengths.

Photoreceptors in the retina of the eye, called cones, translate light frequency into colors. The retina contains three kinds of cones: one for blue, one for green, and one for red. We perceive other colors by combining these colors.

When we see colors, we are actually seeing the effect of light shining on objects. When white light shines on an object it is reflected, absorbed, or transmitted. Glass transmits most of the light that it comes in contact with, and thus appears colorless. Snow reflects all of the light, and so it appears white. A blade of grass reflects green light better than it reflects other colors. Most objects appear colored because their chemical structure absorbs certain wavelengths of light and reflects others.

Black and White

The color black is actually a lack or absence of color. Black, the exact opposite of white light, is the absence of light or the absorption of all light. A black cloth appears black because all the light is being absorbed into the cloth and none is reflected back out.

In the late 1660s, Isaac Newton discovered that white light could be separated into the colors of the rainbow. Newton positioned a glass prism so that the white sunlight could pass through, creating a beautiful spectrum of colors on the opposite wall of a room.

Perhaps an even greater breakthrough for Newton was the fact that he could reverse the procedure and form white light from the spectrum of colors. He accomplished this by placing a lens in the middle of the spectrum to keep the colors of light parallel to each other and placing another prism in the path of the colors. The result was a beam of white light emerging out of the second prism.

Colors

White light is the combination of all colors in the visible light spectrum. When separated from each other, the different frequencies create different colors.

Each color has a particular frequency and, as the frequency changes, the color takes on characteristics of colors next to it on the spectrum. (How might this be similar to us changing our particular signature frequencies?)

Whereas frequencies within the human hearing range may vibrate between 15 and 20,000 cycles per second, light frequencies in the visible spectrum vibrate at more than 100 trillion times per second.

The lowest frequency light is the color red, and increasing frequencies occur as orange, yellow, green, blue, indigo, and, finally, the highest frequency light visible: violet. By the way, this order of colors is also represented in the colors of a rainbow, starting with the low frequency on the outer arc to higher-frequency light on the inside of the arc.

The colors of the light spectrum can be easily remembered by "Roy G. Biv," an acronym for the seven colors.

Chromotherapy

Scientists have studied the effects of color, color therapy, or chromotherapy on our moods, health, and way of thinking for years. When the frequency of color enters our bodies, it stimulates the pituitary and pineal glands. These glands produce hormones, which in turn affect a variety of psychological and physiological responses.

The colors you choose for your apparel and in your environment can have a profound effect on your state of mind and overall health. Some people feel colors. Are you aware of a sensitivity or responsiveness to color? Extraordinarily, color has even been known to have an effect on blind people, who can sense color as a result of energy vibrations created within the body.

> *Color has even been known to have an effect on blind people, who can sense color as a result of energy vibrations created within the body.*

Colors have routinely been used by the "chromatically aware" to energize, reduce stress, and even to help control pain and other ailments. Various colors have different effects on the body. For instance, blue has a cooling effect in hot or humid environments, and is calming and relaxing. Green also has a soothing and calming effect, and is commonly used to help anxiety and nervous disorders.

Red can energize, stimulate, and warm the body. It can help circulation, respiration, and brainwave activity. Orange also has an energizing effect and can stimulate the appetite. Yellow is known as the "mental color," and may help improve the memory and relieve depression.

These forms of chromotherapy may be useful, although discovering your personal color frequencies may ultimately be more effective in achieving vibrational balance than following general use applications. Environmental awareness of your most supportive color frequencies may be used as a modern adjunct to the ancient Chinese technique of feng shui (the art of placement), which in addition to creating vibrational balance, serves to better color your world.

Color Blindness

Some individuals are unable to see various colors due to color blindness, an inherited condition. Many color-blind people do not realize that they cannot distinguish colors accurately. Because a number of those afflicted perceive the color red as green, and green as red, this may be potentially dangerous. Imagine riding with a bus driver who cannot distinguish between the colors of traffic lights or other safety signals!

The first person to discover color blindness was John Dalton, a British chemist and physicist, in 1794. Dalton was color-blind himself and could not distinguish red from green. This condition is known as "red-green color blind." Other color-blind people experience different distortions of colors, and some are able to see only black, gray, and white. It is estimated that 7 percent of men and 1 percent of women are born color-blind.

Though color blindness may not have a direct effect on determining one's signature frequency, it is important to be aware of in terms of selecting the appropriate color placement in one's environment for supporting one's frequencies.

Color pigments have their natural opposites, or polarities. This knowledge can be a useful tool in treating color blindness or when using other color therapies. For example, a color-blind person viewing the color red may see it as green or gray. Or he/she may see the color green as red or gray. This is explained, in part, by the fact that red and green are opposites in color pigment, or pigment-polarities. Other pigment-polarities are blue/orange and yellow/violet.

From the perspective of color therapy, any vibrational imbalances in the body, or its subtle-energy field, could be viewed as a deficiency or excess of particular color frequencies. Using the appropriate pigment-polarity may assist in achieving vibrational balance, as well as aligning one's signature frequency.

For example, if a person is deficient in the color frequencies of red, blue, or yellow, these colors could be used in that person's visible environment for vibrational support. On the other hand, if he/she had an excess of these color frequencies, his/her pigment-polarities of green, orange, or violet would be used. Likewise, any excess or deficiency would be treated with the appropriate color pigment-polarities.

Musical Note-Polarities

The study of color pigments has assisted the development of sound therapy practices designed to enhance wellness and balance one's signature frequency. By determining pigment-polarities, we can now convert these pigments into musical note-polarities.

In music theory and terminology, there is no such thing as a ***note-polarity*** or an "opposite note." However, with the help of color pigment information, we can look at the frequency note associated with a particular color pigment and then view its opposite pigment-polarity. We can then translate this color pigment into its corresponding frequency note, giving us a note-polarity, or opposite musical note.

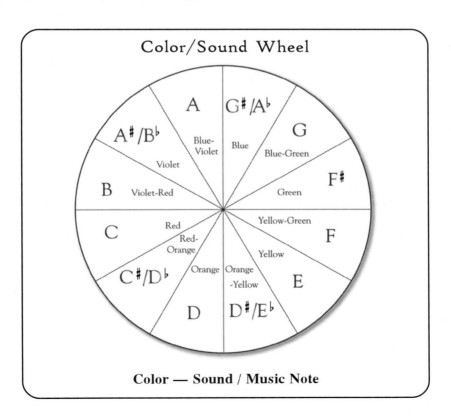

Color — Sound / Music Note

These two previously unidentified, frequency-note-polarities may then be brought into balance in much the same way as the aforementioned color frequency method. In this manner, one could use the appropriate musical note-polarity for vibrational support in one's auditory environment.

The musical note-polarities are as follows: C/F-sharp (F♯); C-sharp (C♯)/G; D/A-flat (A♭); E-flat (E♭)/A; E/B-flat (B♭); F/B. Please refer to the Color/Sound Wheel (page 149) for the colors associated with each musical note.

Note: In this section, when you see two notes separated by a slash, they actually represent the same note. The note is indicated in this manner due to musical notation, which may use either one or the other. For instance, the note of "A-sharp" (A♯) may be notated as "B-flat" (B♭,) or vice versa.

Astrology

When Greek philosopher Pythagoras spoke of "music of the spheres," he was not discussing an abstract concept. He was speaking of actual sounds created by celestial bodies as they moved throughout the heavens. The principle whereby the movement of heavenly bodies influences vibrations is the basis of astrology. Controversy has surrounded astrology throughout recorded history. Its origins date back to ancient times, when astrology was a priestly doctrine used to rule the masses.

> *The principle whereby the movement of heavenly bodies influences vibrations is the basis of astrology.*

In present times, experts in astrology, numerology, and other occult sciences are frequently challenged to prove or defend their positions—unlike professionals in most other fields of study. This is due in large part to religious-based fears, left-brain cynicism, and a lack of substantiating scientific evidence to support the principles that show planetary movements influence personal vibrations. We can accept that the moon and other heavenly bodies can affect the earth, the oceans, the tides, and weather, but have difficulty considering the effects that the planets and stars have on the body-mind.

Thankfully, this rigid thinking is changing as more and more evidence is uncovered by the discoveries of the "new physics" that now supports the tenet that we live in a vibrationally-based universe. This new awareness has prompted scientific research into interesting astrological fields of study, such as "metaphysical" and "medical" astrology.

Music and Physics

In the 1920s, scientist Hans Kayser stated that the whole-number ratios of musical instruments, first observed by Pythagoras, correspond to an underlying framework existing in physics, astronomy, and other natural sciences. Kayser also said that the orbital distance between the planets follows this principle.

The extreme points of the elliptical orbits of each planet remain nearly constant. These constant points were used to create the numeric formulas that constitute the commonly used, even-tempered, chromatic musical scale. Eastern and other ethnic music forms use similar planetary configurations.

The Law of Octaves

Through the understanding of time and frequency, some pioneering astrologers and sound researchers have determined similar tones for the planets based upon the law of octaves. This may have interesting implications for students of astrology and sound alike. The law of octaves states that octaves vibrating at a certain rate and at twice that rate are essentially creating the same sound.

Each individual musical note corresponds to a specific numerical frequency. In the octave of Middle C on a piano, for instance, the note A vibrates at 440 cycles per second. If you move up one octave, the frequency doubles to 880 cps. The next octave of A would be 1,760 cps, and so on, to the top of the human hearing range—around 20,000 cps, or Hz.

Similarly, you can move down in octaves to one half of 440 cps, to 220, 110, or 55 cps, and so on, for lower octaves of the note of A frequency, until reaching the lowest end of the audible range at around 16 cps/Hz. This same method of raising or lowering the frequency, or pitch, can be applied to any note in the music scale.

Brainwaves

Although controversy sometimes surrounds brainwave categorization, brainwave pattern clusters and the harmonics of music are both routinely accepted scientific data. It may be of interest to note that when closely examining the octaves of sound in the lower frequency ranges, they resemble brain wave frequency categories. Examples are shown on page 152.

Could our brainwaves be affected by the vibrations of the planets?

Brainwaves	cps/Hz
Beta	13–30
Alpha	7–13
Theta	3.5–7
Delta	.5–3.5

Octaves Below Middle C	Musical Note		
	A (cps/Hz)	F# (cps/Hz)	C (cps/Hz)
Four	27.5	23.12	16.35
Five	13.75	11.56	8.17
Six	6.87	5.78	4.08
Seven	3.43	2.89	2.04

This correlation between musical notes and brainwave categories suggests that we humans are influenced by the planets and the so-called "music of the spheres" to a greater degree than we may have ever thought possible.

Planetary Frequencies

Planetary cycles are measured in cycles per year, but we hear in cycles per second, so we have to scale up the planetary frequencies a number of octaves to bring them within our auditory range. In this way, we can find specific frequencies and musical notes for each planet and astrological sign.

Some refer to this intriguing area of research as *vibrational astrology* or *astrosonics*, as it refers to the study of the relationship between the motion of planetary and other cosmic bodies and the motion of the earth, rendered as sound vibration. As above...so below?

Notes and Signs

The most popularly studied and used correlations between the musical scale and the astrological signs are as follows:

Astrological Sign	Musical Note	Astrological Sign	Musical Note	Astrological Sign	Musical Note
Aries	C	Leo	E	Sagittarius	G#/A♭
Taurus	C#/D♭	Virgo	F	Capricorn	A
Gemini	D	Libra	F#/G♭	Aquarius	A#/B♭
Cancer	D#/E♭	Scorpio	G	Pisces	B

How do we use this information to further identify, understand, and support our signature frequency? There are several fun and interesting ways in which we can enhance our vibrational awareness through these correlations.

One way is to use tones and music constructed from your strongest planetary influences in your natal chart. Begin by observing which musical notes correspond to your sun, moon, and ascendant/rising signs. If you have other multiple planetary signs in your chart, factor them in as well.

Once you have determined these primary notes in your natal chart, you may use these frequencies individually or collectively in various combinations to support your signature frequency. Some ways of doing this include: listening to sounds, tones, and music that contain your primary notes; toning, chanting, and singing in these notes and keys; and composing musical pieces, songs, and mantras that emphasize your signs, notes, and frequencies.

If you're unfamiliar with music theory, there are composers and musicians who use astrology as a basis for creating personally designed music compositions and soundscapes for the individual. However, unless the creators of these pieces are trained in sound therapy, these pieces may have little therapeutic value. Always use your intuition to guide you in these areas.

Birth-Note-Polarities

Another way of incorporating your astrological information for sound support is by working with your body's polarities. We have numerous polarities within us, which represent dual, opposite, inverse, or reciprocal frequencies. Some of these include positive/negative, male/female, yin/yang, and left brain/right brain. We also have astrological or birthday polarities. Understanding the correlation between your birthday and the associated musical notes will reveal your *birth-note-polarities*.

You can easily determine your birth-note-polarities in the following manner: Find the musical note associated with your astrological sign. Now, count six signs forward, or backward, to locate your polarity opposite (or, you may consult the 12-section Astrology/Color/Sound Wheel on page 155). These two notes, your birth note and its opposite, represent your birth-note-polarities.

For example, the birth note for the sign of Gemini would be "D," the polarity opposite "G-sharp/A-flat," the birth-note-polarities: "D" and "G-sharp/A-flat." The birth note for Aquarius would be "A-sharp/

B-flat," the opposite "E," the birth-note-polarities: "A-sharp/B-flat" and "E." And so on.

Polarity Balance

Knowledge of your birth-note-polarities can best serve you by giving you a focal point for vibrational balance. Sound research has revealed that most people have an imbalance in these polarities. Many unhealthy energies and dissonant frequencies in our living environment—as well as how we react to them—may contribute to these polarity imbalances in our bodies.

Polarity Balance Exercise

An easy way to determine a possible imbalance in your polarities is by following these simple guidelines: As indicated, isolate and listen to your birth note. You can do this by using any acoustic instrument that can resonate your note/frequency, such as a piano, guitar, tuning fork, crystal bowl, or voice. You needn't be trained in music or singing to do this. If you can't sound the note or don't have access to an appropriate instrument, ask someone to play or record it for you.

Next, listen to your birth note for 30 seconds to a minute or so, with your eyes closed, and an intention to resonate with the sound. Notice how you feel. Are you feeling calm, relaxed, and supported? Are you feeling anxious, on edge, and somewhat irritated by the sound? Or do you feel entirely indifferent? When the note stops resonating, do you feel a sense of relief, or a feeling of deprivation?

After assessing your feelings, go through the same process with your opposite polarity note. Again, notice how you feel while listening to the sound. Allow your intuition to guide you. Then compare your responses between the two polarity notes. You will, most likely, notice a difference.

If you feel somewhat uplifted and supported by one of the notes, or you feel a slight sense of deprivation when the note stopped, it's likely that note is weak and needed within your signature frequency. If, on the other hand, you feel a sense of anxiety, irritation, or resistance, combined with a sense of relief when the note stops resonating, then it's likely that the note is too strong, or in excess, and needs to be released from your signature frequency.

Balance is always vital to resonance, healthy polarities, and overall wellness. If, while listening to either of your polarity notes, you feel clear, calm, relaxed, or indifferent to the sound—yet totally present with it—then that note may be in vibrational balance. This is what you're striving to achieve.

Remember that your intention and intuition are the key factors to achieving accuracy in this unique self-diagnostic method for determining resonance in your astrological-birth-sound-polarities and, ultimately, bringing this resonance into your signature frequency.

≈

Is it merely coincidence that there are 12 hours on a clock, 12 months in a year, 12 astrological signs, and 12 notes in the musical scale? The following chart/wheel illustrates the correlations between the 12 astrological signs and 12 musical notes. Also included are the corresponding color frequencies. Note the opposite pigment-polarities and musical-note–polarities.

Although studies thus far have not indicated total accuracy in correlating specific musical note frequencies with corresponding astrological signs, approximately 80 percent accuracy has been reported. This certainly reveals a high enough degree of consistency to warrant serious consideration. And we can expect that one day we may discover more secrets to understanding and using these intriguing astrological concepts for enhanced resonance.

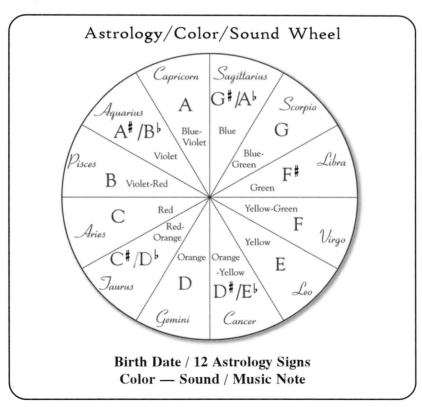

Astrology/Color/Sound Wheel

Birth Date / 12 Astrology Signs
Color — Sound / Music Note

Dowsing

I know very well that many scientists consider Dowsing as a type of ancient superstition. According to my conviction this is, however, unjustified. The Dowsing rod is a simple instrument which shows the reaction of the human nervous system to certain factors which are unknown to us at this time.

—Albert Einstein

Another way to locate any imbalances in your signature frequency is through *dowsing*. Geologists, geophysicists, and physiologists call dowsing the Biophysical Effect Method. With dowsing we go beyond our five senses of sight, smell, taste, touch, and hearing. We journey through the brain wave frequencies of Beta, Alpha, Theta, and Delta and directly access subtle vibrational energy fields for hidden answers.

The word *dowsing* originated in the courts of King Henry VIII. It seems that Henry was desperate to locate stashed treasure troves from pre-Christian kings in order to finance his army. The detective used for this caper was actually the divining hand of a man named George Dowser. From his successful location of hidden treasure, the term *dowsing* came about, referring to finding things hidden underground by using sticks, rods, or plum bobs. Other terms coined to describe this subtle-energy–receiving process are *divining* and the Canadian-based term *questing*.

All three terms refer to the ancient art of locating lost, hidden, or quested-after information, such as objects, people, animals, minerals, or water. Aborigines of various countries have been using "hand dowsing" for water, food, and shelter since the beginning of time.

Dowsing Tools and Devices

Similar to the way radios pick up unseen radio waves, the pendulum or dowsing rod is a powerful antenna that can receive vibrations and frequency waves emitted by people, places, thoughts, and things. There are countless types of tools and devices—natural and man-made—that may be used for dowsing. They are essentially grouped into three categories:

1. **Dowsing Rods.** These are most commonly made from tree limbs and branches, bones, wooden dowels, metals, plastics, or even coat hangers. They are fashioned into swing rods, L-rods, Y-rods, aura meters, bobbers, or antennas.

2. **Pendulums.** A weight hangs on a string, thread, cord, or chain. Some weights commonly used are a gemstone, bead, key, pendant, ring, washer, or needle.

3. **The Human Body.** The body is sensitized and programmed with the intention to feel and respond to subtle-energy vibrations. Some ways in which this can be experienced are body sensations (heat, cold, tingling, tearing eyes, and so forth), gut feelings, "finger responses" (rubbing the thumb and index finger together to detect a yes or no answer), kinesiology and muscle testing, and the use of intuition to access information from within.

Beyond the Senses

Although dowsing is best known for locating water, oil, gold, and other minerals, dowsing devices may also be used for finding lost objects, people, and pets. For centuries, this vibrational process was referred to as "divining," because it involves knowledge beyond the five senses, and was even used in foretelling the future.

> *If you're using dowsing appropriately, you can access information for enhancing your vibrational awareness.*

Dowsing/divining can also be done remotely. This includes map dowsing (water, minerals, lost objects, and persons) and body dowsing (for health issues).

Although the efficacy of dowsing may be difficult to quantify, many successful reports with dowsing have been noted over the years. Based on this success, large businesses and corporations have been known to pay huge sums of money to professional dowsers for locating undiscovered water and mineral resources.

So how does dowsing relate to our signature frequencies? Any time you're working with subtle energy, you're working with frequency and vibration. If you're using dowsing appropriately, you can access information for enhancing your vibrational awareness. This information can then be used to balance your frequencies and vibrational body.

Anyone can learn to dowse as long as he/she has a sincere and dedicated desire to learn. As with most skills, proficiency with dowsing is obtained through practice and experience. However, unlike most other skills, sometimes with dowsing the harder one tries, the further he or she may get from perfecting it. This is because the ego or personality may get in the way of the intuitive vibration necessary for proper dowsing.

An Open Conduit

To achieve success in dowsing, one learns early on the importance of openness, allowance, and being of ego-less service. Begin by allowing dowsing to work through you by placing yourself in a state of passive mental awareness, and then letting the dowsing response occur. Basically, dowsing is in large measure the act of transforming yourself into an open conduit through which information may freely pass.

Next make a conscious request to receive an unconscious muscular reply, amplified by the dowsing tool. When properly practiced, the only effort necessary is simply to relax and allow. Remember that the answer to a dowsing question springs from within. It is an unconscious muscular response that moves the instrument, thus allowing you to interpret the reaction in answer to the question. Therefore, the subconscious mind must be allowed to function, unimpeded by any conscious thought or act.

> *Dowsing is in large measure the act of transforming yourself into an open conduit through which information may freely pass.*

It is important that you remain mentally neutral during the entire dowsing process. Remember that ego, emotions, or extraneous thoughts will interrupt the dowsing signal. If this happens, relax and refocus your attention on your subject. The number of things "dowseable" is infinite and limited only by your imagination. The dowsing language enables us to access information on any subject, anywhere, and at any time.

Yes or No

There are two primary ways to access this information. The first is through accessing the subconscious by asking yes or no questions, and then monitoring the response and movement of the dowsing tool. Before beginning the questioning, however, you must establish what movement represents a yes response, and what represents a no response. Next, establish what movement, or lack of movement, represents a neutral response. (Neutral means neither yes nor no.)

When using a pendulum, for example, the pendulum swinging at any angle or remaining at a standstill may indicate a neutral response. The pendulum swinging forward and backward, or clockwise in a circle, may indicate a yes response. The pendulum swinging from left to right or counter-clockwise may indicate a no response. Similarly, these indications could be used in the opposite. It is entirely up to you to set a clear intention and foundation for a response.

In the same manner, when dowsing with L-rods, decide before you begin if, while holding the rods still, the rods either opening, or closing, will indicate a yes response. Once you've established these parameters, you're ready to dowse.

L-Rods

The other way to access information through dowsing is by the measurement of vibrational energy fields. Because everything has its own frequency wave pattern, we can easily tune in and align with these vibrational auras with dowsing. This is more easily accomplished by using L-rods as a dowsing tool.

Dowsing Vibrational Energy

The L-rods are held one in each hand, chest high, arms relaxed, elbows bent, with the rod tips pointed directly ahead of you. It's usually best while holding the rods, to keep a distance of anywhere from 1 to 10 inches between your hands. The extended rods should be parallel to the ground or floor with the rod tips pointed slightly downward. Be careful they're not pointed too far downward or they will immediately cross. If they're tilted too far upward, they will immediately separate, swinging backward.

Once you have stilled the L-rods and relaxed your mind, stand facing the object or person whose vibrational energy fields you wish to measure. If you have adequate space, 10 to 20 feet is usually a good distance from which to start.

Vibrational Energy Fields

Close your eyes and ask your soul, higher self, or subconscious to indicate the outer perimeter or arc of the subject's vibrational energy field by a movement of the extended rods. As mentioned earlier, the rods may either cross and close, or separate and open, depending on your pre-start intention.

When you're focused, relaxed, and ready—without projecting or expecting any particular response—open your eyes and begin walking slowly toward your subject while holding the rods in place in front of you. At the point of entry into the vibrational field of the person or object, the rods will begin to move and indicate the shift of subtle energy. When this occurs, take a step or two backward, and then again proceed forward to confirm rod movements and note the distance between the subject and the indicated outer perimeter of the energetic field. This distance represents the size and strength of this particular aura and vibrational energy field.

As you become more experienced and adept with this form of dowsing, you may use your L-rods to measure a vast array of energy fields. For space, home, and room clearing, you can use dowsing to detect electromagnetic frequencies, power lines, stagnant energies, entities, and a host of unhealthy or blocked energies. You may also measure vibrational systems in the human body, such as the chakras, meridians, the astral or etheric body, and other energies.

≈

Balance and Support

One of the best ways to use dowsing is in monitoring and supporting imbalances in your signature frequency. This can be easily achieved by first measuring the strength of your vibrational energy field before introducing potentially supportive frequencies, and then measuring it again after. If your dowsing indicates that your vibrational field strengthens and expands with a particular tone, sound, or frequency, then that sound is likely to balance and support your signature frequency. If, on the other hand, your field is weakened and contracted by the sound, then it is likely to be detrimental to balancing your vibrational signature and should be avoided. It may also signal an excess frequency that needs tonal release. This may be further dowsed for more specificity.

To determine if any sound or frequency is beneficial, it is advised to listen to the sound for a few minutes before dowsing, or during the dowsing process. If this isn't possible, the process can work by holding the specific sound-making device—such as a tuned instrument, tuning fork, compact disc, tape, and so on—during the dowsing. Remember the importance of holding a clear intention.

Self-Assessment

Although L-rods are the preferred tool for measuring the strength and size of auras and energetic fields, the self-assessment technique may vary. There are primarily two methods for self-dowsing with rods.

The first method is to face a mirror from a short distance and dowse your image in the same manner as you would dowse another person. The second way is to have another dowser measure your field with the rods.

If you simply require a yes or no response to a question, you may use your L-rods in a similar fashion as you would use a pendulum tool. Depending on how you choose to program them, the rods may expand open to indicate a yes response, for instance, and close or cross for a no response.

Vibrational energy charts are also available to assist in the dowsing process. These charts may offer various guidelines, such as percentages and degrees of measurement for determining specific energetic values.

Dowsing Guidelines

The following basic steps outline the most important points for successful dowsing:

1. Body grounding.
   - ≈ Close your mouth, place your tongue behind your top front teeth, keep your weight balanced upon both feet, and feel your connection to Mother Earth.
   - ≈ Breathe deeply and diaphragmatically to increase and sustain your flow of energy.
   - ≈ Softly tone a deep, low hum or vowel sound.
   - ≈ Drink plenty of water, a good energy conductor, before you begin dowsing.

2. Inner guidance and protection.
   - ≈ Say a prayer or invocation for invoking spiritual guidance and protection.
   - ≈ You may enhance this process by visualizing yourself bathed in and surrounded by white light.

3. Attitude and intention.
   - ≈ Remain open-minded and neutral—mentally and emotionally calm.
   - ≈ Release any projections or expectations about the outcome.
   - ≈ Hold an intention of being in the service of the highest good for all concerned.
   - ≈ Don't try; just allow.

4. Dowsing Process.
   - ≈ Select your dowsing tool of choice.
   - ≈ Follow the specific steps indicated here.

5. Clearing the dowsing tool.

≈ Although some dowsers use soap and water, sunlight, or mental and verbal commands for clearing, vocal toning, and overtoning—fused with intention— are the most effective methods for clearing any object or space. Just focus the sound of your overtones directly into the object or area you wish to clear.

> *Vocal toning and overtoning—fused with intention— are the most effective methods for clearing any object or space.*

≈ Use what feels the most comfortable to you.

6. Programming signals.

≈ Establish your signals—neutral, yes, and no—with the vibrational energy that works in concert with you to respond to your dowsing questions. The vibration is conducted to your dowsing hand, but it's actually your total being that receives the answer.

≈ Note the positions or movements of your dowsing tool by asking for a neutral response, then a yes response, and finally a no response.

≈ Practice asking yes and no questions for which you already know the answer. Once you've established consistent accuracy in your responses, begin creating your own questions to practice.

≈ Continue practicing until you feel confident with the dowsing questions and responses.

7. Framing dowsing questions.

≈ The key to accuracy in getting a correct response is using the right words.

≈ The answer is in the question.

≈ Decide how to word your question.

≈ Be specific. "Does my body need food?" is too general. Be more specific: "Does my body need food at this time?"

Note: Before you begin dowsing, ask your higher self or Spirit if it is the right time to proceed, and if it is for the highest good of all concerned. Dowse for the response. If a no response is indicated, do not proceed further. Try again at another time. If a yes response is indicated, you may proceed.

8. Thankfulness.

≈ After completing the entire dowsing process, offer acknowledgment and thanks to the Divine Loving Consciousness for guiding and supporting your dowsing.

Muscle Testing

Another popular method of dowsing is kinesiology, or "muscle testing." This method of body dowsing can also be used for self-assessment. It is commonly applied by placing a small amount of pressure on a body muscle, arm, or finger, while asking a yes or no dowsing question. After programming the question to the muscle response, a yes answer would be indicated by a strong muscle response and a no answer by a weak muscle response.

> *With the exploration and use of sound, light, color, meditation, astrology, and dowsing, we can better enhance our arsenal of vibrational tools for self-transformation.*

Muscle Testing Exercise

When self-assessing, it is usually easiest to use the fingers and thumbs for a muscular response. Place the tips of your thumb and middle finger together on one hand, and hold them together tightly. Ask a yes or no dowsing question. Using your other hand, try to separate the tip of your middle finger from the tip of your thumb. If the answer is yes, it should be difficult to pull your finger away from your thumb. If the answer is no, they should separate easily.

Another way to do this is to connect the thumb and middle finger on each of your hands, making a "ring" with each hand. Insert the ring of one hand inside the ring of the other like a chain-link. Ask your yes or no dowsing question. If the answer is yes, it should be difficult to the separate the two rings, and "unlink" your hands. If the answer is no, they should pull apart easily.

≈

With the exploration and use of sound, light, color, meditation, astrology, and dowsing, we can better enhance our arsenal of vibrational tools for self-transformation. As we open our right brain's capacity to be intuitively guided by whichever of these subtle-energy modalities resonates with us, we will continue to gather useful information for supporting and tuning our signature frequencies.

(((((15)))))

Sound Relationships

*Approach relationships with the openness of a child, the
perseverance of an adult, and the discernment of the aged....*

—Wayne Perry

When we meet someone for the first time—or even before meeting
him/her—we get a certain feeling or impression of him/her. Some call it a
"vibe," short for vibration. We may feel a "good vibe" or a "bad vibe"
from someone. (Of course, if we feel a bad vibe, it's always coming from
the other person and has nothing to do with us!) Where do these feelings
come from? What role do we play in this "vibe thing?" How does it serve
us? Why are we attracted to some, and repelled by others? Should we
cultivate relationships only with those with whom we feel a good vibe?
Let's look closer at these vibrations.

Chemistry: Complementary Resonance

We've all, at one time or another—often without explanation—felt
uneasy or uncomfortable around certain people. Think back to a time
when you saw or met someone for the first time, someone from whom
you felt a bad vibe or discomforting feeling. Think about that person for
a moment and recall the feeling you had. Now, think of a different person
you met for the first time, when you felt an attraction, a resonance, or
feeling of kinship. Having met neither of these two people previously,
what makes up the core difference in how you felt with each of them?

The answer may be found in the amount of chemistry or ***complementary resonance*** existing between your two signature frequency patterns.
We tend to resonate, or "vibe," with someone who complements our
overall signature frequency. For example, the first meeting involved
your interaction with a person who, likely, had an abundance of a particular frequency of which you had a sufficient or overabundant amount.

This caused a subtle-energy overload, creating a negative feeling within you that you may have interpreted as a "bad vibe." Being unaware of the vibrational principles and interactions taking place can cause us to judge others unfairly, and perhaps, react inappropriately.

Now recall the second meeting with an individual with whom you felt attraction, resonance, and kinship. The subtle energy received was vibrationally supportive. This phenomenon usually occurs when one is weak or deficient in a particular frequency, and another person has a sufficient or overabundant amount of that frequency. In the presence of this emanation, you then feel a positive feeling that you may interpret as a "good vibe." It actually has to do with vibrational polarities and is the essence of chemistry. Sometimes it's mutual chemistry, and sometimes it may be one-sided. But it's all vibrational.

Vibrational Polarities

Opposites do attract. This can be observed in nature as well as in relationships. For example, when in close proximity, positive and negative poles of a magnet quickly and firmly adhere to each other. And conversely, two positive magnets repel each other and cannot be brought together. (Likewise, two negative magnets.)

Similarly, if there is too much "sameness" or similarity between two people in an intimate relationship, there may not be enough vibrational "pull" or chemistry to keep them together. In other words, opposite energies are complementary, generating the vibrational chemistry to attract one another.

This is the principle involved, and is a general rule, but it may also be a simplification when it comes to the complexities of human relationships. For instance, although a potential partner with a completely opposite vibration might offer a strong attraction, an optimal opportunity for personal growth and greater expansion of our emotional experience, we may not be ready for that much growth and change just yet!

Vibrational Impressions

Many factors are involved with how we process our thoughts and feelings about others, particularly during first impressions. The subconscious mind holds many memories and impressions from the past that greatly influence us. For example, we may feel uncomfortable with an individual because he/she simply bears a resemblance to someone who hurt us at one time. We might not be conscious of the resemblance, but the subconscious remembers and reacts accordingly. Perhaps the sound of a person's voice, or their behavior, mannerisms, or style of dress also trigger unpleasant past memories.

On the other hand—and to our possible detriment—we may feel comfortable and secure with an individual who reminds us of someone who was loving and good to us. So many factors contribute to our reactions and receptivity in getting to know someone. Ultimately, we can only know another to the extent that we know ourselves. And when we don't really know ourselves, we often overanalyze our relationships.

You know I think you feel I know you think I feel you know me.

And, I know you think I feel you know I think you feel I know you!

Do all these factors protect or inhibit us from developing potential relationships? Does our trust in those with whom we feel good vibes guarantee us a better chance at a harmonious relationship? Is there a better way of processing and understanding these vibrations? And is there a way of improving our odds in attracting, developing, and sustaining better relationships? I think there is.

Signature Frequencies

Although the many influences within the subconscious mind certainly affect our relationships, the vibrational aspects of relationship chemistry have been virtually unexplored. These aspects are contained within the pattern of our signature frequency.

In conducting voice-analysis-assessments for individuals and couples since 1992, I've observed that, in almost 100 percent of cases, couples routinely have an abundance of the frequency that their partner lacks. This accounts for the chemistry and initial attraction felt within the relationship. However, this can be a double-edged sword. On one hand, there may be a nice exchange of complementary vibrational energy; on the other, a predisposition to co-dependency. The ideal "sonic prescription" would involve balancing and integrating each individual's signature frequency to better harmonize with one's partner for the optimal resonance and development of the relationship.

> *In almost 100 percent of cases, couples routinely have an abundance of the frequency that their partner lacks.*

When Karen first came to my office for a voice analysis, she was concerned that her husband David would discount her belief that they could improve their relationship through enhancing their complementary resonance. Although they had a basically good relationship, Karen felt that their interests were very different and that the chemistry between them wasn't as strong as it once was. She felt they were starting to take each other for granted and that David was less attracted to her. Karen was also concerned that he wouldn't agree to submit to a voice analysis. Fortunately, with a little time and gentle prompting, David came to see me for the voice session.

Not surprisingly, David's analysis revealed a pattern almost identically opposite to that of Karen's. This is quite common with couples, and reaffirms the adage that opposites attract. To sustain the initial attraction, however, it is necessary for both partners in a relationship to grow and strengthen their own areas of weakness within their signature frequency patterns. By instructing them in the use of vibrational principles, I was, thankfully, able to assist Karen and David in strengthening and improving their relationship with each other, as well as with themselves individually. (I subsequently worked with many more couples in a similar manner to assist them in achieving and sustaining improved relationship harmony.)

The most effective way to manifest and sustain a harmonious and fulfilling relationship is by learning to understand and resonate with one's own signature frequencies. With this "vibrational self-awareness," we become better equipped to attract and harmonize with another's frequencies.

Cause and Effect

When we operate unconsciously with regard to the promptings of chemistry-vibrations, we learn our relationship lessons the hard way: being at the *effect* of chemistry, rather than learning the vibrational principles that teach us to understand and embrace the *cause*. By operating from the often painful position of *effect*, we usually find ourselves struggling to hold together co-dependent relationships. When we live at the *cause*, we empower ourselves and each other to take more personal responsibility to thrive in interdependent and harmonious relationships. This signifies the potential of complementary resonance.

If we rise into love, we needn't fall in it.

Dating

In the realm of modern dating services, relationship compatibility is strived for by attempting to match individuals with common interests, lifestyles, looks, personalities, and/or long-term goals for family. The means used have included extensive interviewing and screening, social and religious gatherings, computer analysis, and video or Internet dating. But, when finally bringing the two individuals together through these means, if there is no chemistry between them, there is usually no further interest.

Imagine for a moment the potentialities of a dating service using voice analysis and complementary resonance principles to assist single people in discovering the ideal chemistry in relationships—developing a means to create and enhance a healthy, interdependent chemistry, rather than unconsciously being at the effect of a superficial chemistry. Could this be the "relationship wave" of the future?

You get to the heart of a relationship by relating from the heart.

Sound Relationship Exercise

In 1993, I developed the following exercise for the purpose of enhancing emotional honesty and the development of deeper resonance in relationships. It is outlined in 20 steps, which may be read, one at a time, by each partner in turn. This works best if both partners express themselves from the heart—with open and honest feelings, while maintaining eye contact for a few moments between each step that is read.

Sound Relationships: The 20 Steps for Enhancing Emotional Honesty to Create and Sustain Resonance

1. I remember that there are no accidents, and that everything is unfolding perfectly.

2. I take total responsibility for all aspects of our situation.

3. I agree that nothing you or I am doing is either wrong or right.

4. I realize that each of us is receiving exactly what we want, to teach us exactly what we need to know.

5. I remember that you are my mirror, and however I see you is how I see myself.

6. I also realize that what I experience is how I see the situation.

7. I recognize that the issue is not with you; it is with me. You are a catalyst to assist me in seeing and resolving it.

8. I identify my feelings by being honest with myself about what I'm experiencing, and then resonating with my feelings.

9. I support myself by owning my feelings, yet reminding myself that feelings are not right or wrong, good or bad; they are just feelings.

10. From the deepest feeling level that I am able to express myself, I share with you the complete truth about what I'm feeling in the moment.

11. No matter how you respond to me, I shall do my best to communicate to you from my heart, rather than from my reactive mind.

12. I release all judgments that I may hold toward you, and toward myself.

13. I see any ways that I may be withholding love from myself or from you, and I go behind the apparent circumstances of the situation and locate the love.

14. I feel and express to you that I unconditionally love and support you just the way you are, not how I think you should be.

15. I keep my heart open to you by forgiving you, and by forgiving myself for any pain that I've experienced.

16. I ask your support to see our situation and our relationship in a harmonious light.

17. I resonate with you completely in this present moment.

18. I deeply appreciate your presence in my life and the wondrous beauty of our relationship.

19. I feel the joy that comes when the truth is found and expressed in sound, light, and love.

20. I know resonance and oneness.

Upon completing the steps, you may wish to express your feelings without words, using only sounds, silence, and a hug. (Thanks to Arnold Patent for inspiring this exercise.)

≈

Tantra Toning

There is a popular misconception about or concerning the term *tantra*. Most people believe that Tantra refers to sex, sexual positions, sex yoga, or sustained sexual orgasms. In actuality, out of more than half a million written texts on various Tantra practices and applications, only a small portion of this vast literature makes reference to tantric practices of sexuality.

Tantra developed in India many thousands of years ago and is an elaborate system for applying and integrating the many aspects of vibrational energy: physical, emotional, mental, and spiritual. The word *tan-tra* comes from a Sanskrit root word meaning "to weave" together. This reference to weaving is found in many mystical systems as awareness that all aspects of creation are connected or interwoven, as in a great weaving.

> *The primary purpose of Tantra Toning is to strengthen, revitalize, and harmonize interpersonal frequencies between individuals.*

The philosophy of Tantra recognizes the holistic nature of humankind and the Oneness within, which energizes and connects us. True tantric practices thus emphasize the proper conservation, amplification, and channeling of vibrational energy toward the development of the immortal or spiritual body.

When toning is combined with the integrative power of Tantra, we gain an indispensable tool for personal transformation. We may also use this tool for improving the quality of our personal relationships. Although it may sometimes be used to enhance the sexual experience, *Tantra Toning* is non-sexual in principle, and is a fun and easy way to deepen and sustain intimacy with loved ones. When practiced regularly, it can be very effective in dissolving fear-based blockages that inhibit the natural flow of love and communication between partners. Tantra Toning may be used in all sorts of relationships, including family, friendship, business, and professional, and can also be done in groups.

The primary purpose of Tantra Toning is to strengthen, revitalize, and harmonize interpersonal frequencies between individuals. This empowering process also concentrates and amplifies our complementary resonance. We may then increase awareness and appreciation of our oneness, rather than focusing on separateness and differences within our relationships. Additionally, we raise elements of the body-mind from a lower and denser vibration to a higher and lighter vibration—and from lower chakra stagnation to upper chakra stimulation.

As a sonic meditation process, Tantra Toning may, ultimately, help us to free the soul from the shackles of the gross and temporal physical body.

Couples

To enhance and sustain vibrational harmony and intimacy in relationships, partners may use Tantra Toning for a "dual tune-up" from time to time. The "Gotcher Chakra" toning exercise, as I affectionately refer to it, is an excellent technique for achieving this.

Gotcher Chakra Toning Exercise

Begin by sitting face to face with your partner, close up with your knees touching. You may sit in chairs, or in the lotus position (cross-legged) on the floor or on a bed. To enhance the giving and receiving of energy, place your left hand with its palm up under your partner's right hand (palm-down). Now place your right hand, palm-down, over your partner's left hand (palm-up). Each person's thumbs should now be pointing to their left. Each pair of hands should be touching and resting on the knees, or wherever it feels mutually natural and comfortable.

The next step is to cross-breathe together, inhaling through the nose and exhaling through the mouth. Cross-breathing, in this context, means that when you inhale, your partner is exhaling. And when you exhale, your partner is inhaling. Synchronize your breathing by doing the "relaxing breath" together. (See Chapter 8.) Close your eyes, keep your back relatively straight, and continue breathing together until you feel relaxed, peaceful, and fully connected to one another.

Throughout each step of the process, you may silently communicate your readiness to your partner with a gentle touch or squeeze of the hand.

In the next step, both partners need to focus attention on their fourth chakra or heart center. Breathe deeply into your heart chakra to send energy there.

Imagine a beautiful green light radiating and emanating from your heart chakra. Visualize the light being concentrated into a single beam of healing green light and being projected from your heart chakra to your partner's. Now, see this healing green light being sent from your partner's heart chakra to yours. Strengthen this connection by holding it firmly in your mind's eye and breathing deeply into it.

When you both feel ready, using a mutual squeeze of the hand for indication, gently tone an "AH" sound through the beam of green light to your partner's heart center. Both partners should hold the intention to give and receive sound, light, and love with the toning vibrations created. The eyes should remain closed throughout the process.

After a loving connection feels established, imagine the healing green light expanding throughout your whole body, going wherever it's needed, and then streaming up and out through the crown of your head as if it's a beautiful, glowing green fountain. Allow any energy that may obstruct or inhibit your manifestation and expression of love to be released out through your crown. Affirm that this disharmonious energy be transmuted to a higher frequency. As your partner does the same, you both consciously and vibrationally support each other through each step. After feeling mutually complete, sit together in silence for a few minutes to process and resonate with your experiences.

In a relationship, it's nice to know that your partner has "got your back" or "gotcher chakra"!

Depending on each partner's needs, you may both then move to another chakra requiring attention and support. (For more information on the chakras, refer to Chapter 10.) If this isn't needed, you may complete the process with silent meditation, but always finish with a grounding tone before opening your eyes and discussing your experiences. However, if either of you has any hesitancy or difficulty in sharing the feelings that came up during the process, you may need to work with the fifth chakra to enhance communication.

(**Note:** Whenever doing Tantra Toning with a partner or in a group, it's important to start with the heart chakra for fully opening and allowing the optimal flow of healing love vibrations. Once this step is achieved, you may move to any additional chakras as needed.)

≈

Tantra Toning Exercise

For couples who wish to enhance intimacy during lovemaking, the following Tantra Toning exercise will greatly assist you. After connecting your heart chakras with the technique described in the previous exercise, shift your attention to the second chakra at the navel center. This chakra relates to sexuality, sensuality, and the emotions. Follow the same procedure as previously discussed with the heart chakra, except now use the "OO" toning sound while visualizing orange light emanating from this energy center.

Upon connecting your second chakras, you may now change positions by either lying next to each other, face to face, or switching to the "yab-yum" tantra position. In this position, one partner (usually the man) sits on the bottom with his legs crossed. The woman sits on his lap, facing him, with her legs wrapped around his waist. If necessary, pillows or a wall may be used for back supports. Whether sitting in this position, or lying down, the object is to be comfortable, close, and intimate.

There are no hard and fast rules regarding what you do next. You may wish to connect more deeply by gazing into each other's eyes, sending your partner appreciative, loving thoughts and feelings, or gently caressing each other. Be fully present in the moment. Think only of your partner. Allow yourself to merge into oneness.

When you are both ready, but before any aggressive sexual activity, "sigh" into some deep-voiced tones together. Let the sounds release from deep within you and resonate through your whole body. Keep your voices soft and low for a deep body vibration. Remember to alternate your breathing: One partner is inhaling while the other is toning along with his/her exhalation, and vice versa.

One partner now directs deep tones into a sensually receptive location on his or her partner. Cupping the hands around the mouth and placing them gently against the body will concentrate and enhance the sound vibrations. The volume and focal point may be adjusted until the optimal sensual response is generated. Both partners may lovingly explore each other's bodies with this delightful tantra toning technique.

Tantric lovemaking is not goal-oriented, but soul-oriented.

As the mutual passion intensifies, you may now focus the toning vibrations directly to the genital areas. Have fun discovering which body areas and toning sounds are the most stimulating and pleasing to your partner. Be sensitive to each other's feelings and needs. Communicate through your sounds; try not to use words. Be creative and expressive. But be sure you are interrelating and resonating with each other.

Upon feeling truly connected with your partner, begin listening to the overtones and harmonics within your voices and expand upon them. (Refer to Chapter 12.) With a loving intent, intuitively project various combinations of overtones directly into your partner's body. Allow the sounds created and your partner's responses to guide you. Vibrationally caressing your loved one with this tantra-overtoning technique can assist in creating prolonged pleasure and deep chakra release. With the appropriate intention, these tones can be profoundly healing as well. Explore using these tantra tones with various chakras. Become a sonic adventurer!

Tantric lovemaking is not goal-oriented, but soul-oriented. It ultimately teaches us to let go of ego-gratification and become more aware of the cosmic bliss that lies within all of us.

After a sufficient time, change places and positions, as needed, and allow yourself to receive a similar, loving tantra toning from your partner. Always be patient and responsive with each other. Give and take as much time as is necessary to bond in the unity of sound, light, and love.

The use of Tantra Toning in lovemaking is a wonderful means for creating increased intimacy and sustained sexual resonance. It can also assist us in achieving sublime, spiritual oneness in relationships. Developing the ability to surrender to the Divine Spirit within your partner can facilitate your soul's journey through the body vessel to its Infinite Home.

≈

Healers Gotcher Chakra Exercise

If you work in the healing arts, the Gotcher Chakra Toning Exercise may be integrated very effectively into your healing practice with a few alterations. When facilitating a healing process with a client, determine what issues and chakras are involved, and then follow the initial steps of this Tantra Toning Exercise. Be sure to fully discuss all the steps of the process with your client before you begin, and assure him/her that it is completely non-sexual. Ask for his/her permission before proceeding any further.

The main difference in using this method professionally with a client is this: After establishing a heart connection with the green light visualization and the "AH" toning sound, you must shift the focus of attention to the client's healing issue. You can address the issue by focusing on the physical area in the body where the client is experiencing pain and stress. You may also address the appropriate corresponding chakra and its related body systems and emotions.

Once this is established, it is now important to allow the client to express the sound of the issue, pain, or discomfort. Whether it is physical or emotional, encourage him/her to imagine what the issue may sound like, and uninhibitedly express it vocally. Allow the client sufficient time to feel comfortable in expressing a toning sound that best corresponds to his/her issue. When your client feels safe and supported, he/she can easily tune in to the appropriate sound.

During this process, it is necessary that the sound come from the client, rather than be projected by you. As soon as he/she gets in touch with and expresses his/her sound, however, you may immediately join him/her in vibrational support by approximating his/her toning sound with your voice. This will assist him/her, particularly if he/she is shy or inhibited in expressing himself/herself. Let your client know before you begin that he/she may drop out vocally at any time after you've joined him/her, and that you will complete the sound healing process with your voice. (For more details, refer to Chapter 20.) In my experience using this technique, I find that some will continue to tone, but most will drop out and prefer to just receive the sound. Be sensitive to your client's needs and do whatever works best.

If you are experienced in hands-on, vibrational healing, or are a toning massage therapist, you may wish to put your client on your healing table for deeper work. When working with an individual who has a chronic issue or blockage, you may achieve better results by focusing vocal overtones directly into the appropriate body area. Areas that benefit most by resonating healing sound include the cranium, spinal column, and chest and abdominal cavities, and any chakra in need of clearing and vibrational support. And if it's not personally invasive to your client, any areas of pain or discomfort.

After completing a sound healing session with a client, always remember to clear your energy field with some release sounds.

≈

Toning Groups

Most people who have done toning for any length of time have experienced a toning group. Toning and sounding with others produces many extraordinary benefits. Some of these include:

≈ An environment for practicing and expressing various toning exercises and sounds.

≈ A forum to discuss what may be perceived as personal failures or successes with sound.

≈ Sound support from other toners and kindred spirits.

≈ A group with whom you can share an experience of vibrational healing by giving and receiving sound.

≈ An opportunity to develop sound relationships and friendships with those who will give you honest feedback when needed.

≈   The collective experience of higher vibrational energy, as the whole is always greater than the sum of its parts.

≈   The bonding and enhancement of relationships by experiencing your inner oneness.

≈   Another opportunity to easily access and tune your signature frequency.

≈   Releasing stress and having fun!

Creating a Toning Circle and Sound Support Group

I have hosted a toning circle and healing support group in Los Angeles on a monthly basis since 1991. It has evolved over time, in accordance with the growth and needs of the participants.

As with any group meeting, the better prepared and organized it is, the greater the benefits. Through this group experience I have learned, and continue to learn, much about healing, sound, myself, and others. The following are some tips to assist you in creating your own toning group.

Begin by communicating with those who are interested in participating to determine the approximate number of people, and the space needed to accommodate them. A large group is not necessary and can be difficult to organize in the initial stages. Allow the group to grow and develop naturally. A few committed toners are much more effective than a crowd of indifferent ones. As it is said, "When two or more are gathered...."

Although there will always be some who will be willing to take more responsibility than others, things will flow the most smoothly without a designated leader. If someone always leads the group, or makes all the decisions, dissonance and resentments will tend to crop up. The majority rules. Although certain decisions will need to be made from time to time, it's best if everyone is in service to Spirit as the true leader.

From this perspective, a few questions need to be addressed and some fundamental decisions need to be made: How often do you wish to gather for toning? Monthly? Weekly? Daily? On what day or evening do you wish to schedule your group? How long will each meeting be? Where will the meetings take place? Should the location be regular and consistent, or should it rotate between different locations?

Will it be an open or closed toning group? (An open group is available to all who choose to attend. A closed group is limited to a specific group and number of people.) How formal or casual do you want to make your group? In other words, will you have food, refreshments, socializing, and networking included, or a short, simple meeting with toning only?

From my personal experience, I'll make a few suggestions that may assist you in answering these questions:

≈ Meet at least once or twice a month, or people will lose interest.

≈ If you choose a short, casual meeting, you may wish to meet more frequently. (I have two friends who get up early in the morning and share a brief 10-minute toning session almost every day before going to work.) Whatever best serves the needs of the group.

≈ If you choose a lengthier, more comprehensive group meeting, you may wish to meet less frequently. I strongly recommend, however, that you keep the emphasis on the toning, rather than on discussion, socializing, and so forth. Or, you can keep other activities separate by scheduling time for them before or after the toning group.

≈ Create a safe and unconditionally loving environment for toning and the free expression of thoughts and feelings. However, avoid giving advice to anyone unless they ask for it.

≈ Always let the majority decide issues such as the day, time, and frequency of the meetings, and the location that is most convenient. Most groups meet at someone's house that is easily accessible from everyone's location. It gets confusing for some, particularly new people, if the location keeps changing. So it is advisable to decide on the best site for all concerned. (A regular, small donation to the host is a considerate gesture for hospitality, water, cleanup, and so on.)

≈ Regarding open or closed toning groups, I strongly prefer and recommend an open group. Though I've known of a few closed groups that have worked, for the most part, they are small groups that have attended sound workshops together and are working on specific issues. They prefer the privacy of a closed group to achieve this. With an open group, however, you welcome new people to participate, bringing new energy to the group. You can also be of greater service to a greater number of people with your growing vibrations.

Many underestimate the power of group toning and sound support. Although it is important and necessary to tone individually and privately, we are also social beings by nature and can benefit greatly by vibrational interaction with each other.

Part of the vision I hold for the future is to see toning and sound support groups flourish and resonate in cities and countries all over the world. A network of toning groups could be listed and accessed on the Internet, for example, to enable fellow tone travelers and sound healers to come together more easily and frequently. This can contribute toward bringing humankind to a higher and healthier "human harmonic" for the benefit of all.

> *Toning groups can contribute toward bringing humankind to a higher and healthier "human harmonic" for the benefit of all.*

Group Toning Exercises and Sonic Meditations

There are numerous toning exercises that lend themselves well to a group format, including some that have been previously discussed. What works best are those that enhance listening, creativity, and interaction. The ideal setting would include three or more people sitting together in a circle. The following are some fun and effective group toning exercises you may explore.

Open Toning Exercise

Open toning is probably the simplest and most popular group exercise. It requires a minimal amount of structure and can be done by advanced toners and beginners alike. The basis for this exercise is free and spirited vocal expression. There are no rules, unless you choose to impose them (for instance, no loud screaming). Everyone in the group is encouraged to just let sound freely "play your body." There are no right, wrong, good, or bad sounds—just sounds.

As is the case with most group toning, it works best to form a circle with everyone facing toward the center, eyes closed. You may choose to hold hands, or not. If you do, however, place your left hand facing up and the right facing down (thumbs to the left), for the optimal flow of energy transmission and reception. Breathe deeply and diaphragmatically while reciting the Sound Invocation (see Chapter 16), or any prayer agreed upon by the group. You are now ready to begin open toning.

One or two people may start, or everyone may join in simultaneously. Allow whatever sounds feel natural, fun, and appropriate to come through. They may be relaxing, releasing, or regenerative sounds—including vowels, howls, humming, harmonics, grunts, growls, groans, and giggles. Let yourself be silly, uninhibited, creative, and spontaneous.

Listen to each other and mimic sounds you like. For example, someone may grunt, causing another to grunt a little differently. A third person then giggles, causing others to giggle. Soon, everyone is laughing, and releasing more sounds and inhibitions. Now explore more interesting and adventurous sounds. Have fun. You may do this exercise for only a few minutes, or allow it to go on for half an hour or more. When everyone feels complete, it will stop naturally.

Always allow for a few minutes of silence after the toning has ceased, and close with a grounding exercise before opening your eyes. Take some time to share your experiences with each other.

≈

Group Resonance Exercise

Imagine a beautiful violet flame in the middle of the circle as a visual focal point and catalyst for absorbing and transmuting unwanted energy released by the group. Hold the intention to release, with your out-breath and sound, any dissonant vibration that doesn't serve the highest good of the group.

Focus the attention at your heart chakra. Visualize a beautiful green light radiating from there, and see it expand with every breath you take. Feel it grow and fill your entire physical body, moving through your skin, muscles, bones, and teeth. See this green light filling you up and coming out the crown of your head as though it's a beautiful, glowing, green fountain. It is cascading down, caressing, and bathing your whole body with its healing green light.

When the group is ready, collectively tone an extended "AH" sound from your heart for one complete breath. Release into the violet flame anything that may separate you from your love and healing frequencies, and that could come between you and the group. Ask for these vibrations to be transmuted to a higher frequency. Breathe deeply into your heart space and feel the expanded love and resonance between you and the group.

Allow your attention to now rise slowly upward, as cream rises to the top of milk. Feel it move up through your chest, past your collarbone, and up into the throat area. Focus your attention at the center of the throat and imagine a beautiful blue light radiating from this area. See and feel it expanding throughout your whole body, filling you with its healing blue vibrations. Feel them moving through your lungs, blood vessels, veins, arteries, capillaries, and entire bloodstream. See this blue light filling you up and coming out the crown of your head as a beautiful, glowing, blue fountain. It is cascading down, caressing your whole body with its healing blue light.

Again, when the group is ready, collectively tone an extended "AY" sound from your throat area for one complete breath. Release into the violet flame anything that may separate you from your communication and creativity frequencies, and that could come between you and the group. Ask that these vibrations be transmuted to a higher frequency. Breathe deeply into your throat and heart spaces, and feel the expanded openness and resonance between you and the group.

Allow your attention to again rise slowly upward, as though it's water evaporating into the clouds. Feel it move up past your chin and mouth, through your nose and nasal cavities, settling just above and behind the physical eyes at the "third-eye center." While focusing your attention at this point, imagine a beautiful violet light radiating there. See and feel this light expanding throughout your entire body, filling you with its healing, violet vibrations. Feel them moving through your body, thoughts, feelings, and soul consciousness, as you completely resonate and relax into the present moment. See this light filling you up and coming out of the crown of your head as a beautiful, glowing, violet fountain. It is cascading down, caressing your whole body with its healing violet light.

When the group is ready, collectively tone an "AUM" sound, slowly emphasizing the "AH," "OH," "OO," and "MM" sounds contained within this sacred sound. Tone this sound together for two minutes or so (approximately five or six breaths). As you deepen your spiritual connection within yourself and with the group members, release any remaining vibrational residue or obstructions into the violet flame.

Again, ask that these vibrations be transmuted to a higher frequency. Breathe in deeply through your third eye and fill your entire body with white light, while feeling oneness with the whole group. Sit for a few minutes in silent meditation, resonating with the blissful oneness of sound, light, and love within you.

≈

Group Healing Exercise

Every group member begins by holding an intention about an issue he/she wishes to heal during this process. Follow the initial steps of the

Group Resonance Exercise, except, after toning and opening the heart chakra, shift your focus of attention to 6 inches above the crown of the head. Imagine a brilliant ball of golden light suspended there. With conscious intention, bring the ball of light slowly down, inch by inch, until it enters and merges with your crown. Feel an energizing and cleansing vibration begin to permeate your body.

Continue to bring the golden light down into your whole body, slowly moving through your face and throat, across your shoulders, down your arms and wrists, and into your hands and fingers. See and feel it expanding through your back, chest, and abdomen, and down into your sexual organs, thighs, knees, calves, and ankles, and into your feet and toes. Feel your bones, skin, hair, and every body membrane and system vibrating with healing golden light.

Focus your attention on your body's right side. Project the golden light down your right arm, into your palm, and emanating out through your fingers to the group member holding your right hand. As you visualize the projection of light, consciously send your love and healing vibrations while toning an "intuitively created" sound. Feel the healing sound, light, and love immediately return to you through your left hand, and experience the healing power of group toning.

Now, enhance the healing by switching polarities and repeating the same projection of sound, light, and love through your left hand, to the person sitting on your left. Again, feel the healing vibrations return to you at once, through your right hand. Notice the lessening, or complete dissolution, of your healing issue.

Sit in silent meditation for a few minutes to fully integrate and embrace your healing experience. Offer sincere thanks to the Divine Healer within before completing the exercise with a grounding process.

Many of the toning exercises discussed in other chapters of this book offer wonderful opportunities for group exercises as well, including:

- ≈ **Releasing Sounds Exercises (Chapter 8).** A powerful yet reasonably short exercise for releasing energy blockages.
- ≈ **The Chakra Toning Exercise (Chapter 10).** Due to the expanded vocal overtones and harmonics created by toning vowel sounds with multiple voices, this exercise is particularly beneficial when done in a group format.

≈ **18 Exercises for Creating Harmonics and Overtones (Chapter 12).** These are popular exercises and are highly recommended for toning groups because of their freeform, creative nature.

≈

The Feeling Exercise

The object of this exercise—in addition to having fun—is to assign toning sounds to various feelings. With eyes closed in the standard toning circle format, one person calls out a word and everyone then interprets and expresses it with a related sound. For example, if the word is *funny*, one might make a humorous or laughing sound. With the word *grief*, appropriate toning sounds may include sighing, moaning, and groaning. The word *cold* might evoke shivering or wind-like sounds. You get the idea.

Be creative and expressive with this exercise. It's particularly beneficial for those who have difficulty expressing their feelings. Here's a sampling of some words and feelings that elicit interesting and varied responses: *joy, pain, impatience, lust, fear, love, jealousy, irritation, pleasure, confusion, heat, boredom, anger, heaven,* and *bliss.* Choose your own words, feelings, and sounds with passion and creativity. Have fun with it! Notice which sounds are the easiest and the most enjoyable. Also notice which sounds are difficult for you or bring up resistance. This group exercise can be very insightful and self-revealing.

≈

Group Sound-a-Round

Another fun exercise that develops and enhances creativity with sound, this one usually works best with the eyes open. Someone volunteers to go first and makes a creative toning sound. He/she then repeats it until it becomes very clear and specific. This person then turns to the person on his/her right and passes the sound to that person. The one who is receiving listens attentively to the sound and reproduces it as closely as possible. The original person then drops out. The one toning now feels the sound while repeating it for 20 or 30 seconds. He/she then re-interprets the feeling and sound from his/her perspective.

For example, the first person makes a low, slow "WOW-WOW-WOW-WOW-WOW-WOW" sound, repeating it over and over. The second person first reproduces it, then raises the pitch higher, speeds it up, and alters it: "WOW-WOW-WOW-WOW-MA-MA-MA-MOW-MOW-MOW." When clear and satisfied with his/her sound, he/she passes the sound to the person on his/her right, who continues with the same procedure. Perhaps the next sound expressed is: "MMMOWWW-WILLY-WILLY-OOOPY." Don't be afraid to sound crazy and loopy!

As the sound is passed around the circle (as many times as you like), it changes and develops new tonal dimensions as each individual puts his/her own "sonic spin" on it. When performed with a spirit of adventure, the Sound-a-Round can be a fun and entertaining exercise. It can also challenge you to develop more interesting toning sounds.

Kids usually love this exercise also, as it supports and enhances creative self-expression. Try having some worthwhile family fun with it.

≈

Interactive Improvisation

This can be the most creative and entertaining exercise if participants are willing to release their inhibitions. It is designed to focus and develop communication through sounds, vocal inflections, gestures, and feelings. It's also great fun.

As in the previous exercise, this one also works best with the eyes open. The idea it is to construct an improvised, nonsensical language with tones, vowel sounds, and consonants.

One person begins by getting in touch with his/her feelings and communicating them to another group member, using only sounds—no words. The second person responds similarly, feeling, creating, and expressing his/her own sounds. Although this may initially feel difficult, it quickly becomes easier and more spontaneous as this "sound-speaking" exercise continues. Give yourself permission to sound silly. Imagine that you are speaking some alien or foreign language. Explore the articulation of various sounds and syllables. Improvise and combine them.

Both participants listen to each other and engage in a toning conversation. No standard words should be used—only those that are made up. Add to the dialog by raising or lowering your volume and changing the inflections. Speed up or slow down your vocal delivery. Raise or lower your pitch, abruptly or slowly. Exaggerate your expressiveness. Use dramatic facial and hand gestures. Be creative.

An example of this "jazz talking" or "language improvisation" might go this way:

First person: "CHEE-KONKO, TUBLY-DOH, FEETA-MAY, PO-SNERD-UM, MOOKEE-MOCKEE, RIN-DIL-PERP."

Second person (nodding in approval): "SHNOO-BUTA, SHNOO-BUTA, FLEB-ITY-RAY, CURB-ITA-LAY, MEPIL-TOH."

First person (loudly and emphatically): "VING-GA-TUM, VING-GA-TUM, LA-POON-DEE, LA-POON-DEE. SHI-SHI-LA, TONKA-DOH! TONKA-DOH! SHI-SHI-LA, TONKA-DOH!"

Second person (shaking head and putting hand up): "MEE-KA-POH, SNOO-KEE, SNOO-KEE, FLEE-BA-NOM. MOY-YUNG-GUL, FRIP-PINGLE, EEE-SUM-POOLY-POOLY!"

First person (looking frustrated and asking a third person in the group for support): "SHIB-LEE, SHIB-LEE, ROP-RUNA, KA-BLUNA! CHUM-DELLA-PEW, BEELA-TONKA-DOH, TONKA-DOH! FLURBITY, MURBITY, KREEN-DOPPY-YOPPERS!

Third person (joins in, softly): "YOMINY-YOMINY, ZEE-BEKLE, PITZIL-FRITZIL, MOOM-ME-SHLIP, RIFF-EL-ZIP."

Perhaps a fourth person joins in and responds with impatient sounds and gestures. A fifth person then contributes loving and nurturing sounds to all concerned. The group continues spontaneously and creatively as long as desired.

≈

Sound Relationships are a choice; they are not created by chance. They are birthed from self-love, grown with commitment, strengthened in the service of Spirit, and sustained by conscious awareness.

We can know, love, and resonate with another, only to the extent that we know, love, and resonate with ourselves. The level of self-honesty we practice within ourselves will reflect the level of honesty we are capable of with others. The healing principle for Sound Relationships states:

> *Sound Relationships are a choice; they are not created by chance.*

≈ My relationships will manifest and develop in accordance with the clarity and specificity of my intentions.

≈ My relationships will be successful in direct proportion to the agreements and commitments that I make and keep with myself and others.

≈ My relationships will thrive and sustain in an atmosphere of love and devotion to the Infinite Soul that is within each of us.

We must learn to love and embrace all of humankind—not just with lip service, but with all of our hearts. It is a vital part of our life's purpose, because each person in our life represents and reflects a part of ourselves. As we learn to love each and every part of us, through accepting and loving others, we come into resonance with ourselves.

> *We can know, love, and resonate with another, only to the extent that we know, love, and resonate with ourselves.*

Everyone is our mirror. If we feel dislike or hatred for another, this teaches us that we are judging and withholding love from a part of ourselves.

If you hate a person, you hate something in him that is a part of yourself. What isn't a part of ourselves doesn't disturb us.

—Hermann Hesse

As we learn to truly see, accept, and love ourselves, we begin to see more love in others. We ultimately come to the realization that we are all one—many individuated parts of the same Whole. When we see this Wholeness and Oneness within ourselves, we can't help but see it within everyone. It becomes impossible not to love them.

However, as with everything in our physical and finite reality, this love is illusionary. From a spiritual perspective, we really can't love anyone but ourselves. When we feel that we love another, we are really loving ourselves in their "illusionary presence." Or you could say we are loving an individuated part of our Self. We may experience the "illusion of the many," but in spirit we are One. One Lover. One Beloved.

For example, if you pressed all 10 of your fingertips against a steamed-up window, we would see 10 fingerprints on the glass. The illusion is that they were made from 10 separate objects. From a larger perspective, however, we see that the 10 impressions were made by only two objects: your two hands. And, from a still larger perspective, we can see your two hands are connected to only one body.

> *We may experience the "illusion of the many," but in spirit we are One.*

Similarly, by expanding our ego-based perspective of the "separated self" to the unifying awareness of the "One-Spirit-Self," we enter a new paradigm in understanding the Infinite Relationship.

PART IV

Vibrational Healing With the Voice

Much like an opera singer may shatter a crystal wine glass by singing a high, sustained note, similarly, the power of vocal overtoning can shatter subtle energy blockages in the body which can cause tension, stress, pain, and may lead to disease.

(((((16)))))

Your Core Keys: The Eight Principles of Healing

Before we can best use our innate healing power in concert with the guidance offered us by universal healing principles, it may be useful to closely examine our therapeutic tools, or what I call "core keys." Once you find your core keys you'll seldom lose track of them again (providing you use them). These foundational key principles lie within each of us and are important to recognize and understand in order to maximize our effectiveness in sound healing, creating self-transformation, and voicing our souls. Some of these core keys are simple and basic in concept and will be summarized concisely. Others, due to their more comprehensive natures, will be explored in more detail.

The first of these keys is in many ways the most important, because it expands the power and efficacy of the others. Think for a moment about what might be your most powerful and valuable attribute or function of consciousness. Which aspect of your human awareness that you use daily has the most impact on your personal experience of life, as you perceive it? Is it your mind? Your senses? Your thoughts or feelings? Intuition or creative energy? Sense of humor? Your passion, compassion, or capacity to love? Is it your voice? Your spirit?

These are all good answers. However, I would submit that there is one attribute we all possess that empowers and amplifies all of the above—a natural aspect of our consciousness that illuminates everything we perceive and energizes everything we say or do. This attribute and function of human awareness is our attention. This is our first core key principle.

1. Focused Attention

Tell me to what you pay attention and I will tell you who you are.

—Jose Ortega y Gasset

When you pay attention to something, you shift from passive to active awareness. This activity focuses—and thereby energizes—your awareness. There is tremendous energetic power in focused attention. As Deepak Chopra and others have stated: Where attention goes, energy flows. This points to the ability in human consciousness to concentrate and direct the flow of awareness between the body-mind and its experience. And in proportion to the quality of attention—and clarity of intention—it creates both the transmission and reception of vibrational energy.

> *The mere act of focusing our attention participates in creating reality moment by moment!*

Quantum physicists have confirmed in the laboratory that in classical tests, the act of observing the experiment alters the results of the experiment. Remarkably, when we put our attention on a quantum field, sub-atomic particles such as quarks, bosons, and neutrinos come into existence. When we are not placing our attention on the field, these particles are just a probability amplitude in the field of infinite possibilities.

These particles are so small that there are no instruments available to measure them. So if we can't measure them, how do we even know they exist? We actually know this by the evidence of the trails they leave behind in particle accelerators. This quantum field phenomenon means that the mere act of focusing our attention participates in creating reality moment by moment! Could this lead us to understanding the secrets of creation?

Quality and Quantity

How we use our attention certainly seems to create the circumstances and outcomes of our lives, and ultimately defines who we are. According to Deepak Chopra, M.D., in *Ageless Body, Timeless Mind*, "The quality of one's life depends on the quality of attention." For example, if we want to be successful at something, we must put attention into it. If something is important to us, we're likely to put more attention into it. And if something is life-threatening, it gets our full attention. Similarly, negative results may be observed because what we focus attention on expands. If we inappropriately put too much attention into something, it tends to disrupt and dominate our lives. A compulsive gambler puts too much attention on gambling. An addict puts too much attention on the addiction. A workaholic focuses too much on the job. Even a person who puts too much attention on his/her family can be controlled by family, if attention isn't properly put into meeting individual needs and responsibilities to oneself.

Think also about how valuable and important your attention is to others. Just walking or driving down the street, you can see signs and billboards designed to capture your attention. Turn on the radio or television and there's someone trying to get your attention. Newspapers, magazines, e-mail, junk mail—before they can get your money, they need the most valuable thing you have: your attention!

Those of us who have children know that they need almost constant attention; the elderly do, as well. Your attention is the vehicle for expressing consciousness and love. It is the most powerful crystallization of your soul's human awareness—and everybody wants it!

"Attention" Journal

For a reality check, I suggest keeping a journal for at least a week, to keep track of where you are placing your attention each day. How much attention goes into work, family, friends, study, relaxation, leisure activities, and so forth? Write it down; note the hours and minutes you devote to each of these concerns each day. Be honest with yourself—it may surprise you.

> *As you learn to harness and discipline the energies of attention, healing abilities will increase proportionately.*

How does the focus and distribution of your attention affect and reflect the present state of your life? How much time do you give to yourself each day? What quality of attention do you put into your own personal growth, needs, and development? How much time and attention do you give to the Inner Spirit and your soul? To what or whom are you giving the most valuable thing you have? Within the answers to these questions lie the secrets to peace, personal power, sound health, and true freedom.

Give your attention to the Almighty Power that is giving you life and strength and wisdom.

—Paramahansa Yogananda

In the realm of healing, incredible results have been created with the help of focused attention, because it concentrates the vibrational energies transmitted through consciousness. As you learn to harness and discipline the energies of attention, healing abilities will increase proportionately.

Because your attention expands the energy of that which you focus upon, it's important to be mindful of what you want to expand. For example, if you focus your attention on your pain, disease, weakness, or fears, they may expand and become worse. If, on the other hand, you focus on appreciation for the lessons they brought to you, or on your strong and healthy components, then those are the factors that will expand. As you practice this shift in attention, attitude, and consciousness, you'll experience the true value of mastering focused attention.

The material universe is nothing but the "self" experiencing itself through various qualities of its own attention to itself. If your attention is divided, then you are divided. If your attention is on fear, you are fearful. If your attention is on love, you are loving. If your attention is on wholeness, you are whole. If your attention is on Oneness, you are One.

By the way, thank you for giving me the most valuable thing you have!

2. Prayer/Invocation

A vital core key to healing and transformation is to acknowledge and invoke the True Source of our being. By aligning ourselves with this Divine Spirit, we allow the grace and power of the Infinite One to permeate our finite, individuated selves with limitless potentials. And, because the abundant grace and love of Spirit is always present within us, we need only invoke and evoke its presence by being an open conduit through which sacred sound, light, and love may flow.

Drawing on your religious beliefs, faith, or spiritual orientation, you may use any prayer or invocation that you resonate with to facilitate this intimate connection. The most important aspects, however, are to simply be sincere, open-hearted, and specific about your intention.

If you haven't a favorite prayer or invocation to use, you're welcome to use the Sound Invocation that I have created and developed over the years. It is designed to be very specific and empowering for the purpose of invoking the sacred and healing flow of Divine Source Energy.

The Sound Invocation

I invoke and evoke the Divine Loving Consciousness
of the Infinite Spirit within me.
I am a clear and open channel for Sound,
Light, and Love.
May the Sound of Light uplift me.
May the Light of Sound guide me.
May the Love of Spirit embrace and protect me.
May the Sacred Sound of my Soul now resonate through
me for the healing and harmony of all.

3. Conscious Breathing

The power of breath, the central breath,
attracts from space all the different elements
which are there...all that one can get
from an herb, flower or fruit and even more.
Therefore the breath can achieve a thousand
times more than what medicine can do.

—Hazrat Inayat Khan

The breath—often taken for granted, yet an extremely powerful element in our therapeutic repertoire—is referred to in the East as *prana*, or life force energy. When understood and used properly, this core key is a phenomenal tool anyone can use for healing and transformation.

Conscious breathing involves using focused attention in concert with the life force energy of the breath to effect a specific intention. When you direct a healing intention through the breath and into a particular body system, you infuse that system with the supportive vibrational energy of consciousness. You can most effectively use this key principle by directing your breath into that which you want to release, transform, or heal. If it is a physical issue, breathe directly into that body system, organ, muscle, body part, blockage, or pain. If the issue is emotional, the principle is the same; simply breathe into that feeling or emotion to facilitate the necessary healing in that system.

Tips

When consciously breathing, some tips to remember are:

≈ Close your eyes (unless you need outer vision—while driving, for instance) and feel the breath coming through your nostrils, into your lungs, and then moving directly to the body area in need of healing energy.

≈ Continue this breathing process until you experience a relaxing or releasing feeling in the targeted area.

≈ Allow your body to release any blockage, resistance, or unhealthy energy, via your exhalation.

≈ Develop a more conscious and intimate relationship with your body by practicing this breathing method regularly, as needed.

≈ Breathe diaphragmatically. (Refer to the diaphragmatic breathing exercise in Chapter 7.)

Pulsed Breathing

One of the most important conscious-breathing techniques for facilitating healing work is *pulsed breathing*. Through the use of pulsed breath we can release blocked or unhealthy vibrational patterns and make room for resonant, healthy ones.

Pulsed Breathing Exercise

There are two ways to use pulsed breathing for clearing and releasing undesirable energy patterns:

1. **In-Pulse Breathing.** While closing your mouth, draw in short, forceful breaths through your nose while contracting your abdominal muscles. Continue emphasizing multiple in-pulses of nose-breathing between gentle nose exhalations.

    In-pulse breathing is primarily used for the withdrawal of vibrational patterns needing healing and transformation. This technique is most frequently used in doing healing work on others.

2. **Ex-Pulse Breathing.** Inhale deeply through your nose and hold it for a second or two. Then forcefully ex-pulse your breath, through the nose, while contracting your abdominal muscles. Repeat several times.

    Ex-pulse breathing is best used in combination with release sounds, as it facilitates clearing your body of dissonant vibrational patterns. Ex-pulsing your breath can be a most effective self-healing technique for releasing unwanted thoughts, feelings, stress, pain, or even other people's vibrations that may affect you adversely.

    ≈

> *Through the use of pulsed breath we can release blocked or unhealthy vibrational patterns and make room for resonant, healthy ones.*

When we clear or release something through pulsed breathing, we free ourselves of its influence over us. We change the "form" of a thought or feeling by energizing or de-energizing its vibrational pattern. For example, with in-pulsed breathing we withdraw so much energy from its structure that it can't sustain itself and collapses as if it were a deflated balloon. On the other hand, with ex-pulsed breathing we project so much energy into the structure that it can't contain it all and explodes, as an over-inflated balloon might.

As we practice conscious breathing techniques, we better facilitate the healing process—triggering the vibrational energy that moves us through inner and outer transformation—toward our desired reality.

Nose or Mouth?

A question I'm often asked by my students is: "Is it better to breathe through the nose or the mouth?" There are different opinions about this, but to keep it simple, I recommend the following: If you feel tired, sleepy, or fatigued, *mouth-breathing* is best for supporting optimal wakefulness, alertness, and energizing. If, on the other hand, you feel restless, anxious, on edge, or impatient, then *nose-breathing* is preferable, as it will assist you in calming down, relaxing, and being more present. However, if you feel present and in balance—neither fatigued, nor anxious—simply inhale through the nose and exhale through the mouth. This is the best breathing method when you feel grounded, centered, and fully present.

Before beginning any healing work, remember to check in with your feelings and notice how you are breathing. Then—still breathing diaphragmatically—select which of the three breathing modes best supports you in the moment. Keep in mind that you can always shift between them as needed. There is much to be gained by breathing consciously.

A note to parents: You may notice that when children feel fearful, anxious, or impatient, they breathe quickly and heavily through the mouth. The best way to get children to settle down and relax is for them to breathe through the nose. (The trick is getting them to do it!)

I'm sure you've heard the expression "it takes all kinds." Well, I've never met any kind of person who doesn't breathe! We should be appreciative for the wondrous gift of this life force energy.

Breathing through all the pores of life is the one Life.

—Paramahansa Yogananda

4. Inner Listening

Opening ourselves to hear and feel sound is ***inner listening***. Rather than limiting our hearing to receive sound only with the ears, with inner listening we intuitively open ourselves to listen with our bodies, feelings, and higher selves.

The essence of this important listening principle involves the ability to transcend the environmental influences and social programming that condition our feelings and reactions to various sound input. As we shift the focus of attention from our outer awareness of sound to our inner experience and responses, we begin to develop a more intimate relationship between our body-mind and our signature frequency. This inner listening practice leads us to listening with the soul.

Inner listening leads us to listening with the soul.

In our usual listening mode, we tend to stand apart from a sound and analyze, judge, and categorize it—whether consciously or unconsciously. This separates us from the full experience of it. It may also be a self-protection mechanism. With inner listening, though, we actively involve ourselves more experientially with the energy of the sound, so as to gain more comprehensive information and potential healing benefits.

For a better understanding of this core-key principle, it may be helpful to observe the three different ways in which we receive and process sound. The first is through what we call hearing, a passive function. We can consciously or subconsciously hear many sounds simultaneously. While listening to a speaker, for instance, we may hear someone else in the room talking or moving. At the same time, we may hear other noises in the room, such as a fan, a heater, an air conditioner, clinking glass, or rustling papers. Also, there may be sounds coming from outside: traffic, music playing, a barking dog, the wind, or rain. Because this mode of hearing is more passive, our attention may drift between some or all of these sounds, while still hearing the speaker.

The second way we receive and process sound is an active function: listening. When we withdraw our attention from the sometimes distracting sounds that we passively hear, and focus our attention on a particular sound or voice, we are then actively listening. The listening mode of processing sound concentrates our awareness so that we may absorb more information for learning retention. However, because the functions of focusing and retention vary according to the individual—and not everyone learns and retains information in the same manner—there's a third mode of processing sound that can maximize reception and retention. This is what I refer to as intuitive or inner listening.

In his book *Being and Vibration,* Joseph Rael states:

> A true human is a person who knows who he is because he listens to that inner listening…. Inner listeners, or people who are continually listening to life as it is unfolding, are

true humans because they are picking up vibrational messages before the messages become crystallized energy or
perceptual forms that can then be articulated by the brain....
In that process of listening, the voice of guidance is found.

Sound Listening

Unfortunately, most people don't truly listen. For example, while listening to someone speaking, we can be so quick to react emotionally to
what we think we are hearing, we don't truly hear what's being said. This
may be similar to how we listen to sound. If a sound or a piece of music
immediately feels unfamiliar, harsh, erratic, or too loud, we often react
negatively or with resistance. We generally prefer things that are "easy" to
listen to, relaxing, or pretty. Our ability to be open and receptive to sound
frequencies is shaped by many factors.

In terms of sound healing, this puts us at a disadvantage. For instance,
it may not be a pretty or pleasing sound that can effectively break up and
release an energy blockage, such as a kidney stone or tumor. It is helpful to
release our expectations about the way sound should sound and give ourselves an opportunity to truly experience it. Rather than quickly judging,
resisting, or reacting to what we think we hear, when listening to words,
sounds, or music, what may better serve us is to keep our focus of attention on ourselves—examining how we are feeling and why. This is a more
conscious and resonant way to listen. It's actually intuitive, inner-listening,
and a form of sonic meditation.

To learn how to better listen and resonate, let's examine some of the
root factors that may block or negatively influence our responses to various
sounds:

- ≈ **Mood:** mental or emotional state of listener.
- ≈ **Predisposition:** genetic/social/environmental.
- ≈ **Incompatibility:** with signature frequency.
- ≈ **Volume:** degree of loudness or intensity of sound.
- ≈ **Pitch:** tonal range of sound (low/high).
- ≈ **Tempo:** speed of rhythm, beats, meter (fast/slow).
- ≈ **Tonal Quality:** texture of sound (smooth/abrasive).
- ≈ **Constancy:** continuous or repetitive sounds.

≈ **Dynamics:** variation and contrast in force or intensity.

≈ **Dissonance:** discordant sounds.

≈ **Source:** type and quality of sound reproduction.

≈ **Sensitivity:** to the subtle energy and intent behind sound.

As you begin to recognize the circumstances and factors that are unconsciously inhibiting your inner listening capabilities, you can shift your attention accordingly.

Noise Pollution

Another issue of concern, which may be helped by the practice of inner-listening, is that of noise and sound pollution. Many people are more concerned with food, water, and air pollution, but awareness is rapidly growing of the dangers in various sound frequencies that pollute our environment. Research has shown, for instance, that those who live in close proximity to elevated sound levels, such as airports, have higher levels of stress and a greater incidence of cancer and heart disease. Some work activities have also shown, over time, to have harmful effects on the body. Some of these include working in noisy environments such as factories or playing in loud rock bands.

We may be doing irreparable damage, not only to our hearing, but to the entire body-mind. Although the best remedy may be moving to another location or changing jobs, this is not always practical or possible.

One of the most effective ways I've found to create a positive sound environment with inner listening is by using the Noise Pollution Exercise (page 199). This is a popular exercise I developed some years ago to assist in combating the deleterious effects of sound pollution. Before entering into the active, inner-listening portion of the exercise, you may begin by identifying which types of sound or noise you find the most disturbing and annoying. This is a subjective issue and will not be exactly the same for everybody. For one, it may be the sounds of a leaf blower, subway train, motorcycle, or jackhammer. For another, the sounds of a siren, dog barking, crying baby, or yelling voice. To still another, the subtle hum of electricity, a refrigerator, air conditioner, or a constant water drip. Think about it: Which sounds bother you the most?

After feeling complete with recalling the various sounds representing the most disturbing noise in your environment, you're ready to move on to the next step. Think about how you would define noise. What exactly represents noise to you? What are its characteristics? Does it involve volume? Tonal quality? Is noise simply sound that is distracting or irritating? Is it associated with constancy or repetition? With invasiveness or surprise? Is the most upsetting noise connected to your past or childhood? Give yourself ample time to reflect on these questions and how these sounds may impact your life.

A New Definition

Once you've come to a better understanding of what noise represents to you, you may find it beneficial to consider a new definition. Allow yourself to think, for a moment, about a more responsible and empowering perspective on defining noise. The definition that I choose to embrace is as follows: *Noise is a value judgment of a sonic experience.* Is that too simplistic? Not realistic? Doesn't the word *noise* inherently infer that upon its entering our perceptions, the sound of it has some control over our thoughts and feelings, thereby making us its victims? Have we turned over our power to this merciless sonic oppressor? Is there a possible escape from the relentless clutches of this torturous vibration? Relief is in sight—or, shall we say, "in sound."

> *We may do more damage to our health by resisting noise than by listening to it.*

Granted, as mentioned earlier, there are circumstances in which noise or sound—whether in the audible or inaudible range—may have damaging effects. However, in the vast majority of circumstances, there is much that we can do to protect ourselves from unhealthy sound. This can be a controversial topic when taken out of context, but in most situations—and this is important to understand—we may do more damage to our health by resisting noise than by listening to it. Again, the old adage "what we resist, persists" is apt.

Noise Pollution Exercise

So, let's move on to the more active part of the Noise Pollution Exercise. The first step—after affirming that noise is simply a value judgment of a sonic experience—is to "inner-listen" to the imposing sound. This means that rather than trying to block out or resist the sound, you fully receive, listen to, and resonate with it. In this way, you begin the process of shifting from being at the effect of the sound experience to the position of being at the cause of your experience.

Next, with your eyes closed (when appropriate), imagine the sound moving up and through your body, unobstructed, and being released through the crown of your head. Breathe deeply into the sound, facilitating an acceleration of the release. Then tone the sound just the way you hear it (don't try to create the perfect sound effect; just reflect how you feel it), emphasizing any vowel sounds with increased volume for optimal releasing. Finally, lovingly bless the sound and release the process, while creating a feeling of appreciation for the gifts of resonance and the lessons learned.

≈

Inner Listening Exercise

At perhaps the opposite end of the spectrum, a listening exercise for gaining the most benefit from healing sounds, regenerative sounds, vocal sounds, or music is the Inner Listening Exercise. Close your eyes and diaphragmatically breathe into the sound, thus fully engaging the life force energy within the breath. Next, imagine your whole body as one big "sound sponge" or reception device. As you envision yourself listening with your skin, bones, and hair, as well as with your feelings, senses, mind, and soul, this engages not only your ears, but also your full, holistic resonation capacity. Are we not more than a physical body? Let us resonate fully and use all that we have available to us in human consciousness. This is true inner listening.

> *Stop the mental jabbering. Still the mind. Be fully present.*

To optimally support the process, you should consciously affirm staying in the present moment throughout the listening experience. Joseph Rael said in *Being and Vibration*: "Listening is understanding the mystery of vibration because listening has to do with the inner vibration of the descending intelligence of the moment." Control any mental tendency to be distracted by the past or future. You needn't ponder what occurred earlier in the day, what you have to do later, how long the process will take, and whether you are doing it right! Stop the mental jabbering. Still the mind. Be fully present.

Finally, you need to give yourself conscious permission to receive sound—and this can be profoundly important for some. We often don't take the necessary time to give to ourselves, especially in the healing arts. You need to allow yourself the opportunity to fully receive and be supported. This may sound simple to some, but oftentimes people have difficulty in this area—feeling that they don't deserve to receive. In fact, we all deserve to receive the healing blessings of sound. We need to give ourselves—and others—the gift of listening.

Sound is a carrier wave of consciousness, and, when we learn to trust it, we find it always goes where it's needed. Likewise, trusting our intuition leads us to what we truly need. By simply opening our "resonant receptors" to its many blessings, we can experience the profound healing power of sound through inner listening. And it's great to resonate!

≈

5. Visualization

We should learn how to visualize our thoughts—how to recharge them with the energy of concentration until they become visible manifestations.

—Paramahansa Yogananda

Visualization is the act of making something visible by forming a mental image. Visual pictures and mental images enhance communication between our perceptual, emotional, and physiological functions. As a result, when combined with sensory input and vocal sounding techniques, visualization can enhance emotional clarity, expand healing energy, and create profound effects within the spiritual levels of self-awareness.

> *There is great energetic power in our capacity to visualize, for it leads to creative manifestation.*

Although similar in principle to our previous core-key inner listening, visualization employs our focused attention on visual, rather than auditory awareness. There is great energetic power in our capacity to visualize, for it leads to creative manifestation. If, as quantum physicists have demonstrated, our mere attention can affect the state of matter, then we can begin to imagine the possibilities of creating new realities with visualization and the limitless potentials of consciousness.

If we can imagine it, we can create it.

Man can only become what he is able to consciously imagine, or to "image forth"

—Dane Rudhyar

Visualization Exercise

In a healing context, there are two basic aspects to using visualization. The first involves recognizing the issue you want to heal and holding a specific mental image of it, just the way it is. The second aspect involves re-imagining, re-creating, and re-patterning the issue, or body system, and seeing it in its natural resonance and healthy state. Understanding these two aspects of visualization will assist you in shifting your focus from any resistance you may have around the issue, to envisioning what you want to create, and then manifesting it.

An exercise to better facilitate the process of visualization for healing is as follows. Close your eyes, and with your inner awareness, hold a mental picture of the issue—body system, organ, emotion, pain—that you want to release, transform, or heal. If it is not physical, use your imagination to find an appropriate form or symbol that will represent the feeling within the issue. For example, a feeling of sharp pain might be visualized with the symbol of a sharp object, such as a knife; a feeling of loneliness could be symbolized by a sole, wilting flower; a blockage in the body could be viewed as a dam. Allow yourself to be creative with your visualization. (It will become easier with practice.)

Next, breathe deeply and directly into this form or mental image while visually defining it more clearly with each successive breath. Imagine and use any associated forms, such as shapes, colors, and backgrounds, if they better assist you in focusing your clarity and attention. Be as specific as possible with your visualization.

You can't depend on your eyes when your imagination is out of focus.

—Mark Twain

You may now use your visualization energy and intention to transform the old form into a new form that better serves you. Allow your imagination to re-create and manifest the optimal healing results. For instance, you may see blocked or stagnant energy shift into vibrant, flowing energy; diseased cells and tissues regenerate into healthy ones; dense or contracted forms transform into open, expansive ones; heavy darkness burst into brilliant light; clashing colors and shapes blend into complementary and harmonic ones; painful or repressed emotions blossom into joyous, loving ones; or limited beliefs expand into limitless possibilities. Visually re-patterning the form in consciousness facilitates the manifestation of your desired intention and is a powerful tool for transformation.

Because what you focus your attention on expands its energy, it's important to use caution with regard to how you shift from the unhealthy issue to the healthy one. In other words, spend more time visualizing the new, healthy, resonant energy rather than the old, unhealthy, dissonant energy. Complete the exercise by seeing the new feeling or body system filled and resonating with healing, vibrant light.

Conversely, there have been numerous studies in subtle-energy medicine indicating that even positive affirmations may expand illness and disease—including cancer cell growth—by placing too much attention on the disorder. There are also healers who make the error of trying to attack, kill, or destroy a disease. This is a mistake. As you learn to honor and respect all life forms, you begin to realize that everything has its perfect purpose and place in the Universe. All you need to do is simply trust, and act from love rather than fear. And remember to put enough time, energy, and focused attention into healthy, harmonic visualizations for the best results.

> *When you add visualization to the toning process, you create an end result for the sound.*

When you add visualization to the toning process, you create an end result for the sound. By imagining both the sound and form of a particular body system, you can better heal and transform it. This unbeatable combination of vibrational energy can dramatically enhance your effectiveness in achieving mind-body harmony and wellness.

≈

6. Entrainment

Entrainment is universal in nature…. It is a physical phenomenon, but also is more than that, because it informs us about the tendency of everything that vibrates—in other words, everything—to swing together, to lock in. It informs us about the tendency of the universe to share rhythms, that is, to vibrate in harmony.

—Joachim-Ernst Berendt

The World Is Sound: Nada Brahma

Originally discovered in 1665 by Dutch scientist Christian Huygens, **entrainment** is the locking in step of rhythms. It is a process of mutual phase-locking, whereby the natural rhythms, frequencies, or vibrational patterns of one object are actively changed by the vibrations of another object.

Rhythm is an aspect of sound. Each rhythm or pulse of sound creates its frequency, which is measured in cycles per second. The phenomenon of entrainment, with its periodicity of countless rhythms and cycles, can be observed throughout our living environment. There are daily cycles of dark and light, changing seasons each year and corresponding cycles of harvest, and mating and gestation cycles and patterns.

Nature Rhythms

Every form of life has its own unique rhythms and cycles that determine its habits and characteristics. For example, insects such as bees, hornets, and locusts fly in swarms; schools of fish swim together, almost as one; geese fly together, locked in a V-formation. In the past, scientists thought this was due to a leader with more intelligence or experience. Now we know these habits are directed by entrainment.

Stronger rhythmic vibrations affect weaker ones, causing them to lock in step with the more dominant ones. A unique demonstration of the phenomenon of entrainment was conducted by filling a room with various grandfather clocks and setting their pendulums in motion at different intervals. Although all the pendulums would initially swing differently from each other, after several hours, all the pendulums were found to be swinging together in perfect synchronization. (We performed a similar experiment during a sound healing workshop I conducted in Pittsburgh some years ago. During the lunch break, we placed some clocks and all of our wristwatches in a bathroom. After the workshop concluded that evening, we checked the clocks and watches, and found all their second hands ticking and moving in sync together.)

Other examples of this entrainment process include the transmission and reception of frequencies generated between radio and television sets and broadcast stations. On old sets in particular, when you adjust the knobs, you are adjusting the frequency of your set's oscillators to align with the frequency of the station's oscillators. When the frequencies come within a certain range of each other, they suddenly lock in, or entrain. When musicians improvise or "jam," they almost telepathically tune in to a particular rhythm or chord change. They are entrained with each other. Ministers and their congregations entrain with each other, as do professors and students, or two people engaged in deep conversation. Groups of female college roommates will often have their menstrual cycles at the same time after one or two months of living together. All of these occurrences reflect the principle of entrainment.

Body Rhythms

As we observe some of the normal functions of our bodies, we can easily notice the rhythmic patterns in our breathing, talking, and walking. For instance, we don't usually speed up and then abruptly slow down our voice while speaking. There is a natural rhythm, meter, and flow to the speaking voice that is uniquely individual. Likewise, when we walk, we don't combine short, fast steps with long, slow ones (that is, unless we are a member of Monty Python's gang!). Each individual has his own rhythm and gait.

We also have cycles that determine the body's sleeping, eating, digesting, eliminating, and respiratory and heart rate rhythms and patterns. Within the body, blood cells—when interacting with one another—suddenly change their rhythm and start pulsing together in perfect synchronization. Our heart rate, respiration, and brainwaves all entrain to each other, and their frequencies all function harmonically.

> *Music and sound therapy can slow down brainwaves, thereby affecting heart rate and respiration.*

Our bodies are constantly locking in our own rhythms to better resonate and function physically, mentally, and emotionally.

Notwithstanding that the various functions of the body-mind can entrain to each other, it is also possible to utilize external rhythms to affect and activate internal body functions, such as brainwave activity. Music and sound therapy have been shown to slow down brainwaves, for example, thereby affecting heart rate and respiration. You can also slow down your brainwaves and heart rate by slowing down your breath. This all points to the healing power available to us within sound and entrainment.

Brainwave Entrainment

Brainwaves are rhythmic electrical waves of the brain and can be affected with sound waves. This process, called *brainwave entrainment*, involves creating special rhythms and pulse rates that cause a sympathetic response in the brain. Entraining brainwave states can effect remarkable human change and growth, such as increased creativity, super learning capabilities, focusing of attention, behavior modification, sleep induction, pain control, relief from stress, increased memory, and dramatic improvements in mental and emotional health.

According to Dr. Jeffrey Thompson, director of the Center for Neuroacoustic Research:

> Brain wave entrainment is part of a larger biological function called "Biological Sympathetic Oscillation." Our biological clock sets itself to external cosmic events; day length cycles, full moon cycles and seasonal cycles, to name a few. The body will set itself to the most powerful external pulse cycle it is exposed to. In this case we can create powerful sound frequencies pulsing at exact brain wave speeds and cause the brainwaves to alter themselves to match the sound frequencies—that is, entrain themselves to the sound pulses, thereby altering one's state of consciousness.

There are a number of techniques available for the support of brain functioning and brainwave entrainment. Some of these methods include beat frequencies, waveform phasing, Hemi-Sync, binaural beats, sound wave pulsing, treated music recordings, and vocal overtoning practices and recordings.

A rudimentary knowledge of brainwave patterns and their related states of consciousness may assist us in better understanding the value of entrainment to enhance mind-body wellness. If we can use sound waves to change brainwave rates and cycles, we can use sound to change anything else that vibrates. And everything vibrates.

Frequencies

There are various ways in which sound and entrainment have the ability to affect the pulsations or frequencies of the brain and the body. For instance, some years ago, while studying various sound research, I discovered that two slightly out-of-tune frequencies would cause the predominant lobes of the brain to change their rhythmic patterns and entrain to the difference between these two frequencies. For example, if the first frequency was 50 Hz, and the second was 60 Hz, the difference would be 10 Hz. This third frequency, or "difference frequency," could then be used to create sounds for changing the brainwaves.

I subsequently learned that the brain was also affected by a fourth frequency in the previous example. This was the sum of the two original frequencies, or 110 cycles per second. So, in addition to the original 50 Hz and 60 Hz frequencies, also produced is a very low 10 Hz (below the hearing range) and a much higher 110 Hz. This multiple-frequency phenomenon (called *heterodyning* in old radio jargon) has important significance in sound therapy practices. These multiple frequencies, when used appropriately, can create some of the most healing and regenerative sounds available to us.

Though used in conjunction with therapeutic techniques ranging from sound machines to music therapies, the most effective use of multiple frequencies may be with the natural harmonics and overtones of the human voice.

Because vocal patterns also reflect brainwave patterns, the technique of voice assessment is a common sound therapy diagnostic tool. A deficient frequency indicated in the voice, for instance, may correspond to a body system deficiency indicated in the brain wave pattern. Upon determining which frequency is deficient in the brain wave pattern, the frequency can be introduced in the form of a specific sound, pitch, or musical note. With repeated listening to the note, the brain will eventually entrain to that frequency and begin to create it on its own, enabling the body to heal itself. The frequency will also return to the voice. This sound entrainment process has been shown to effectively strengthen and improve previously weakened body systems.

In much the same way that a song we hear on the radio may stick in our mind after repeated listening, a needed "nutritional frequency" with similar repetition can stick in a way that offers us therapeutic benefit. For example, if you are deficient in a brainwave frequency of 32 Hz, it would correspond to the musical note C. This note or frequency can be applied in any number of different octaves by simply multiplying it by 2, or dividing it by 2: 16–32–64–128–256 (the frequency of middle C). Any of these frequencies may be used individually, or in various combinations as multiple frequencies. You may also use the same principle for any other note or frequency.

We can gain greater insight into how we are routinely affected by sonic entrainment by noticing the way songs, jingles, and pieces of music stay in our mind. We may often sing, hum, or whistle these catchy "sonic slices" of music, but do we understand their significance in how and why they affect us? What is their relationship to entraining our brainwaves?

Recall for a moment a song or melody that stuck in your mind. If possible, try to remember the first time you heard it. Once you've recalled the familiar melody, answer the following questions: How many times did you hear the song before it stuck in your head? Is it a song or jingle that you like, or one that is irritating? Why did that particular melody stick with you, and not most others you heard?

What answers do you come up with? Many factors may influence our responses to a song or piece of music: listening volume, repetition, type of music, our mood, memories, and past associations. However, a virtually unexplored factor in this response mechanism is that of our signature frequency. A primary reason for your entraining with, and therefore remembering, a particular piece of music may be that it is compatible with and supportive to your own vibrational needs.

You may not even like the piece of music you are recalling, but your brain is dispassionate and is automatically drawn to any frequencies it needs. It may be a simple radio or TV jingle that you can't seem to get out of your head. It may sound silly or obnoxious to you, but there's something in it that appeals to your brain, and your body probably needs some frequency in that jingle. It might be the music key, the primary note pattern, the harmonics created, or the rhythm—whatever it is, you're entrained by it.

Notice also the importance of repetition in this entrainment process. We seldom, if ever, sing or hum a melody after hearing it just once. It's only after repeated listening to a piece—usually three to four times or more—that the tune or melody entrains itself in our memory. This shows us that entrainment is a passive function of the brain, and we needn't sit down and try to memorize a sound pattern. We need only hear it repeatedly. Repetition is a key factor in sonic entrainment.

Other sound patterns or pieces of music may contain overabundant frequencies that may be incompatible with your signature frequency. These sounds or melodies may be forgettable and flow in one ear and out the other, as they are unlikely to be needed by your brain or body. However, if you are overly sensitive to sound—and are not familiar with intuitive listening practices, such as the Noise Pollution Exercise (page 199)—these excess frequencies may feel invasive and irritating.

Of course, this is not an exact science (yet), and sometimes we are drawn to sounds and frequencies that are not necessarily supportive of our vibrational needs (similar to how some are drawn to foods, substances, and people that are not healthy for them). However, the more time we spend learning, understanding, and using the principle of entrainment, the more we can empower ourselves. We can then choose sounds, songs, music, tones, and frequencies to entrain our brains and bodies with the optimal resonance and vibrational support.

Remember: Entrainment demonstrates how weaker vibrational patterns are affected by stronger ones. It's not difficult to imagine the incredible possibilities available to us for strengthening weakened body systems with entrainment. The human body has a natural ability to entrain and heal itself when it is supported and allowed to do so. Entrainment with sound is another powerful core-key principle that we can use as a vibrational therapy to support and transform body wellness.

7. Intention

In order to achieve a particular outcome or result, it is important to have a concentrated, deliberate, and clear intent. In healing work, the specificity and clarity of our intention is vital. In his book *Ageless Body, Timeless Mind*, Deepak Chopra states, "Intention is the active partner of attention; it is the way we convert automatic processes into conscious ones." And elsewhere he says, "Attention focuses awareness to a local perception. Intention brings about a change in that localization." So when we consciously combine the core-key principles of attention and intention, we create a powerful foundation and vehicle for transformation.

Intention and Imagery

Remarkable healing results have been achieved with the use of intention. In his book *Healing with Love,* Leonard Laskow, M.D., states:

> In a series of experiments I found that, with imagery alone, I could induce an eighteen percent inhibition of tumor cell growth in culture relative to controls. When I included the intention for the rapidly growing cells to return to the natural order of their normal growth rate together with imagery of reduced cell growth, the inhibitory effect was doubled to forty percent. In these studies it seems that imagery and intent each contributed equally in influencing the psychoenergetic inhibition of tumor cells in culture.

Irrespective of the context, our intent is the energy that drives activity and shapes our results. For example, if we have an intention to build a house, we need to first look at all of our prerequisites: finding the ideal location, surveying the available land and property, deciding on size and design, determining costs, financing, and any other issues of concern. Next, we would need to obtain the necessary permits and licenses, blueprints, materials, tools and equipment, workers, and any other supplies needed to proceed with the construction. In time, the needed building components, combined with the clarity of our intention, will result in the creation of our house.

> *Our intent is the energy that drives activity and shapes our results.*

The healing process is no different. Upon deciding what we wish to release, transform, or heal—with a clear intent—we can implement and use all the core-key principles as our tools, materials, and supplies for building our "human house," our "body temple of resonance." Intention is the focused energy within human awareness that brings our efforts into crystallized, manifest form. When this energy is fused with sound, light, and love—our primary essence—the growth and healing potentials are limitless.

Consciousness

While exploring various subtle-energy healing modalities throughout the years, I've often been perplexed as to why seemingly contradictory practices can achieve similar results. Sometimes, for example, a particular healing sound for pain release may work successfully for one person and have no effect on another. The latter may derive similar pain relief from a completely different sound. How can this be? I've come to the conclusion that the key lies in one's consciousness, beliefs, and intent. Because of the infinitely shifting and transformational nature of consciousness—and each individual's signature frequency—intention cannot be easily quantified.

When we consider the use of sound with intent, we are ultimately looking at the consciousness of the sound being created. Is there a difference between our conscious and unconscious intent? If we are feeling conflicting emotions while putting out an intention, do those emotions affect our intent? I believe they do. Because we're dealing with different aspects of energy, all of these consciousness issues are inextricably intertwined. And because sound is a carrier wave of consciousness, these issues need to be considered—particularly when they involve healing.

One way to better understand our own possible duality of intention is to observe how we experience others. Think about how you may be affected by another person's voice when he/she is speaking to you. Do you feel the sincerity of his/her conscious intent, or do you feel a different message in his/her tone? When you watch a great actor, or listen to a creatively talented singer perform, can you feel the present-moment power of his/her intention—even if the sound of his/her voice is raspy, or leaves something to be desired aesthetically? On the other hand, can you feel a lack of intent and presence in a performer who possesses a trained and extraordinary voice? By using inner listening, we can learn that the difference is in the consciousness encoded into the intent and voice. This example illustrates that one's conscious intention is more powerful than the actual sound being created.

Healing Intention

The following exercise contains five questions to better facilitate the use of intention for self-healing. It works best if you take sufficient time to think about your responses and then write them down. After you've explored your thoughts and feelings by writing, condense your answers into a few sentences. Start from the awareness that all of life is a transformational process and that all healing is self-healing. Accept that healing is possible and that you have a choice. To consciously heal, you need to gain access to what you want to heal, and then form a clear and specific intent to do so.

Healing Intention Exercise

Preliminary Healing Questions

1. *What do I want to change, transform, or heal?*

   What circumstances, symptoms, feelings, thoughts, attitudes, or beliefs do I want to release or change?

2. *What is prompting me to change, transform, and heal at this time?*

   Is the desire to heal and transform coming from within me or from external sources? Here you are identifying your motives for changing.

3. *How did or do I see myself as contributing to the present circumstances?*

   In this question you are looking for how the choices you made in the past, or are presently making, contribute to the circumstances you want to change. You are not looking for blame or fault. Rather, your goal is to identify your choices and beliefs so that you can literally choose once again. Realizing that you had and still have a choice shifts you back into the seat of your power.

4. *What does having this issue, illness, or situation keep me from doing, having, or being?*

What does it now allow me to do, have, or be? What might I be gaining from this issue? How has this situation changed my life? What is the payoff I am receiving from the circumstances?

5. *What result or outcome do I want to create?*

Where do I want to go from here? If I knew that in whatever I tried I could not fail, what would I do? What would I have? How would I be? What do I really want? What is my destination on this journey? What brings me joy and fills me with love? What is my bliss and ecstasy? Here you address the meaning of your true desires, your intention, and sense of purpose.

≈

These questions will assist in clarifying your intentions and give you an opportunity to review your past, present, and future. They start to seed the subconscious in preparation for healing work. Although they may not lead to immediate answers, to the extent that they are honestly addressed, the answers will sprout in the soil of psycho-vibrational interaction and contribute to the creation of a fertile environment for the growth and development of your healing.

> *The easiest instrument through which intention can be focused and directed is the human voice.*

In terms of sound therapy and vibrational healing, the easiest instrument through which intention can be focused and directed is the human voice. It is the most immediately accessible tool we have available to us, and when we use the voice—whether for ourselves or for others— we automatically focus on the present moment in creating a healing result. My colleague, Jonathan Goldman, frequently states his formula: "Frequency + Intention = Healing." This means that the intention of the person working with the sound is as important as the frequency used to create resonant frequency healing. I believe this to be so; it may even be more important, because the intention always holds and reflects the consciousness of the healer.

The simplest and most effective way to achieve results with intention is to remember our second core-key of prayer and invocation, and hold the intention of being an instrument of Spirit as a vehicle for sacred healing sound. As we align ourselves with this humble attitude of service, we create the best environment for clarity and wellness to manifest. This may be our purest and highest intent.

8. Commitment

Put your heart, mind, intellect and soul even to your smallest acts.
This is the secret of success.

—Swami Sivananda

A commitment is a voluntary act of giving one's energy, attention, fidelity, skills, time, and word to someone or something specific. To commit oneself involves making a conscious and trusting connection with an ideal, a cause, or a purpose, or with another person or persons. Perhaps the most important commitments are the ones made with ourselves. If we're not committed to our own highest good, in integrity with ourselves, it's impossible to truly commit to others or anything else.

My face is set, my gait is fast, my goal is Heaven, my road is narrow, my way is rough, my companions are few, my guide is reliable, my mission is clear. I cannot be bought, compromised, detoured, lured away, turned back, diluted, or delayed. I will not flinch in the face of sacrifice, hesitate in the presence of adversity, negotiate...at the table of the enemy, ponder at the pool of popularity, or meander in a maze of mediocrity. I won't give up, shut up, let up, or slow up.

—Robert Moorehead

We have all known people with the best of intentions who never seem to follow through with them. This demonstrates a lack of commitment and points to the necessity of committing to our intentions, to ourselves, and to others. Intention without clarity, commitment, and follow-through leads nowhere. The results of our intentions will be in direct proportion

> *Partial commitment doesn't work. We either commit ourselves totally or not at all.*

to the agreements and commitments that we make and keep with ourselves, and, in turn, those made and kept with others.

We should never underestimate the power within our thoughts and words, for not only do they display the nature of our character, but they can also sabotage the results of our intentions if we do not follow through with commitment.

If you don't make a total commitment to whatever you're doing, then you start looking to bail out the first time the boat starts leaking. It's tough enough getting that boat to shore with everybody rowing, let alone when a guy stands up and starts putting his life jacket on.

—Lou Holtz

One of the difficulties we have with making commitments is that we often feel guilty about failing to honor previous commitments we have made. Our intention behind commitments needs to be about the present, rather than the past or future. We need to renew a true commitment in every moment of every day. In this manner, past, present, and future merge into the present moment, and we thereby honor and fulfill our commitment.

Partial commitment doesn't work. We either commit ourselves totally or not at all. Mastery of life demands 100 percent commitment. Ironically, total commitment can be easier than a halfhearted effort. Someone once said, "99 percent is a bitch—100 percent is a cinch!"

Another problem many of us have with commitment is that we confuse commitment with a relinquishment of personal power—particularly in the context of relationships, in which we trust another person with a part of ourselves. Due to previously experienced emotional pain and fears, we become convinced that the other person will have control over our lives.

> *Commitment is to intention as sunlight is to a flower.*

The truth is that we can commit only to ourselves. Another person is just a reflection of the state of our own consciousness. We are always viewing and experiencing various aspects of ourselves. Committing to ourselves is an act of self-love—and is essential for any healing to take place. The quality of love that we consciously hold for our Soul Self will determine the results of our intentions.

By understanding and practicing this level of commitment, your intentions will fully blossom in the light of love. Commitment is to intention as sunlight is to a flower. With the nurturing, loving light of commitment, your intention will bloom beautifully and purposefully.

Commitment leads us to the most vital and powerful of all healing principles: love. Because of its multidimensional nature and infinite potentials, it deserves its own chapter. So, turn the page and fall—or arise—into love.

(((((17)))))

Love: The Ninth Principle

*Love cures. It cures those who give it
and it cures those who receive it.*

—Dr. Karl Menninger

Love is the most powerful vibration in the Universe, and the most transmittable frequency available to us. Any thought, feeling, or information conveyed with loving energy will create a greater effect than any other energetic transmission. Because of its all-pervading capacity to serve as a multidimensional vehicle for information, love is the most potent of all healing vibrations.

*It is only with the heart that one can see rightly; what is essential
is invisible to the eye.*

—Antoine De Saint Exupery, *The Little Prince*

Resonance

As discussed earlier, every form of matter is composed of energetic vibrations unique and natural to it, which make up its signature frequency. When a form or object is vibrating in a way that is characteristic to it, it is said to be in resonance. When one object vibrates at the natural frequency of another object, resonance occurs.

> *Love creates an energy field that affects all who enter it.*

This principle may be observed when you strike a guitar string or a tuning fork within close proximity to another guitar string or tuning fork that shares the same resonant frequency. Even though it has not been struck, the second instrument will begin to vibrate sound merely by being in the same energetic field as the first instrument. Thus resonance is a cooperative interaction between two objects that share the same frequency.

Similarly, love creates an energy field that affects all who enter it. Within the influence of a strong loving field, if there is the intention for healing to occur, the body's innate, self-healing capabilities will be amplified and enhanced. In the process, we use love to heal ourselves and support others by releasing energy patterns of separation, and resonating with energy patterns of wholeness.

The desire and pursuit of the whole is called love.

—Plato

One word frees us of all the weight and pain of life:
that word is love.

—Sophocles, 406 BC

When we see love as a harmonious energy pattern of universal resonance, we begin to recognize love as a powerful vibration that can influence all other frequencies to shift into wholeness and healing. Through the power of love, we can heal and become whole. With loving feelings, actions, and expressions, we can experience our universal relatedness and Oneness.

Although love has many expressions, its essence is relatedness. In *Healing with Love*, Leonard Laskow, M.D., states, "Love is the awareness of relatedness and the impulse toward unity.... What you can love, you can heal. Love in this sense is the universal harmonic."

When a body system is in the state of wellness, it is creating a resonant frequency that is natural and harmonious with the rest of the body. When disease occurs, however, a disharmonious energy pattern is created in that body system. Through the use of sound and love being projected into the diseased system, energy patterns can be re-established, returning the body to its state of wellness through the principle of resonance.

What's the answer? Loving. What's the question? It doesn't
matter; the answer will still be loving...the first word in healing,
the antidote to stress, the ease that dissolves dis-ease, the Magic
Bullet of Joy, the vaccine against hatred, the positive action we
can take when negative thinking flares, what we can always be
grateful for, proof positive that the blessings already are, the heart
of forgiveness—Loving.

—John-Roger

A State of Being

Love is not logical. It is a state that transcends reason, and its purpose is to allow the experience of a vast shared reality. Love isn't a feeling; it is a state of being. It is changeless. Love asks no questions and makes no judgments or demands. It is always flexible and gentle. It is always unfolding, extending, embracing, enlightening, and expanding beyond all limitations. When we choose the resonance of love we rediscover that peace, harmony, and wellness are our natural heritage and state of being.

> *When we experience true love, we don't fall in love—we stand in love. We stand for love.*

Love, and all things shall be added unto you.

—Jesus Christ

Being in love is not the same as having fallen in love. When we experience true love, we don't *fall* in love—we *stand* in love. We stand *for* love. When we fall in love, an opening is created for repressed feelings to surge forth and attach themselves to another person. We are deluding ourselves when we believe that another person is who or what we love. The other person is but the reason or pretext we have for allowing ourselves to feel love. Only we can choose to open or close our hearts.

Conditional Love

Falling in love is conditional love, a projection onto our loved one of our idealized image of him or her. In reality, our attraction to the other person is basically our attraction to our own projection. Conditional love is but a weak imitation of the vibration we experience in unconditional love. When we love another because he/she meets our needs, we are loving conditionally. When we give love to get love, similarly, we are placing conditions on our love. Although most of us may have grown up with and learned this model of love, once we taste the pure nectar of unconditional love, we instantly become aware of its pristine and transformational qualities. We learn that we can never be truly fulfilled by settling for conditional love, for it is not true love.

Unconditional Love

Love cannot be concealed once it has entered a person's heart.
He may not speak it out but his eyes reveal it.
Once love enters a man's heart it keeps him happy at all times,
for he then becomes free from worries,
and a current of love flows out from him automatically.

—Kabir

True love fulfills itself by naturally flowing out to what is loved. If love returns, it is a gift and a blessing, but it is never required, expected, or demanded. True love is always unconditional and expresses the innate harmony of the Universe. This limitless love has a universal frequency capable of resonating with all others. In a state of unconditional love, our awareness evolves as we grow to value, love, and heal ourselves. We then begin to resonate with others through a new array of interactive vibrations. In the resonance of unconditional love we can experience the heart-filled joy of infinite relatedness with our **True Being**.

> *True love is always unconditional and expresses the innate harmony of the universe.*

Love is a decision and commitment. To love is indeed costly. To love unconditionally is a life wager. In love we put ourselves on the line and there's no going back. It is at this brink that so many seem to collapse. Within arms' reach of greatness, they faint at the thought of never returning. It is the less-traveled road.

—John Powell, *Unconditional Love*

Unconditional love stimulates within us and evokes the deeper, spiritual qualities of love characterized by resonances such as selflessness, forgiveness, forbearance, compassion, gratitude, joy, humility, devotion, and heartfelt service to others. This limitless love roots out and dissolves all fear—the primary impediment to the full realization and experience of love. In aspiring to unconditional love we hold the purest of intentions. In his little gem of a book, *Love Is Letting Go of Fear,* Gerald Jampolsky, M.D., says, "Fear cannot exist in the presence of love. Love cannot exist in the presence of fear. Love is letting go of fear... Love will enter into any mind that truly wants it, but it must want it truly."

We Go Back a Long Way

Reborn of longing
our souls returned to love
We said, "Forever,
we'll be together...."
We go back a long way
to a life we left behind,
When you touched me with your spirit
and I kept you on my mind.
We go back a long way,
so we can make love last
If we remember the future,
we can heal the past.
We said, "Forever,
we'll be together...."
We said, "Forever...."
We said, "Forever...."

—Wayne Perry, *Remember the Future*

I Love You

I can recall a profound moment of insight into the nature of love while attending a lecture at the University of Chicago in the 1970s. The presenter was East Indian philosopher Ishwar Puri, who spoke on Spiritual Mysticism. During his presentation, Mr. Puri made the following statement regarding love: "So many songs, poems, and books contain the phrase, 'I love you,' innumerable times. People's verbal expressions, countlessly, say the same thing, 'I love you, I love you'—frequently, without sincerity, commitment, and true consciousness." Mr. Puri later went on to say, "When we say, 'I love you,' we are, in effect, putting our self (I) first and the beloved (you) last." Then he profoundly stated, "If we truly love someone, we would instead say, 'Love you I,' thus putting the spirit of Love first, and our self (I) last, in the deepest and purest expression of love." Those words resonated and have always stayed with me.

Love You I

As a singer and songwriter, I wanted to write a song evoking this unique perspective on expressing love. Over the years, I tried many times to put these sentiments to words and melody with little success. I was always too much "in my head" about it and couldn't quite keep it as simple and pure as I felt was necessary to let the spirit through, so I gave up trying to write it.

Over time I often thought about this unique view of love, and worked hard in my personal life to transform the quality of love in my relationships. Then in spring of 1998, a few months before my daughter's impending wedding, I was inspired to write a special song for the occasion as a gift to her. I was overjoyed by her invitation to sing at the wedding ceremony.

Around this same time, I had just started recording my fourth music CD, *Remember the Future,* the theme of which was "healing with love." Late one evening after returning home from the recording studio, I found myself still feeling energized and started humming a melody that seemed to be coming through me. Almost immediately after that, words started "popping out." They fit the simple melody perfectly—a "marriage of music and words" graced with love. "Love You I " was finally born!

After some tweaking and arranging, I lovingly performed it—through many tears—at my daughter's wedding, and subsequently decided to record and include it on my CD. My gift for my daughter had come back to me and blessed me with love many times over.

> "I love you" doesn't say,
> Love comes first. So today,
> Before me—you will be.
> I'll tell you why—
> Love You I
> "I Love You" people say,
> But for me it's not the way.
> Love comes first, so I say,
> "Love You I, Love You I...."

Self-Love

We must accept and love ourselves before we can truly love anyone else. As the popular song goes, "Learning to love yourself is the greatest love of all." This is an inspiring sentiment, but there is a popular misconception regarding self-love. To totally empower and free ourselves, we need to love our True Self, the pure Soul Self. We begin by accepting and nurturing ourselves, but it is not "self-centered" love that expands and liberates the soul—it is "self-surrendered" love. We need to surrender to Infinite Love. As we merge with the Infinite Loving Vibration within us, we become free from all separation and ultimately become One with our True Self. This transcendent awareness of our Oneness leads to a state of ecstasy and bliss, a result of the highest consciousness and the purest state of love: Divine Love.

Divine Love and Devotion

Love is the inherent quality of the soul.

Love is the sustainer of life. Just as a lotus lives
on the water, its growth is in the water and it blossoms
through the currents of water in it. Similarly,
love is the life of the soul, and the existence
of the soul is dependent on Love of God. The soul
becomes happy when love takes hold of it.

Love is that which transforms the small drop
of the soul into the ocean of God.

—Huzur Maharaj Sawan Singh Ji

The Philosophy of the Masters

The experience of unconditional love, Oneness, and Divine Love awakens within us our innate capacity for loving service. The purest act and expression of loving service is that of devotion, or Bhakti. Devotion to our True Self, or God, is the highest form of service.

Loving devotion to our True Self is also the greatest commitment we can make to our highest good. We begin to see others in the same light as well—thus deepening and strengthening all our relationships, because we see the Divine Essence in everyone.

Love and devotion, though not exactly the same thing, sort of "hold hands." Devotion is a more subtle yet no less important expression. Although it may be a higher ideal, the concept of devotion is foundational to the topic of love.

I have gained valuable insights and understanding of how we grow into love and devotion by observing the five types of devotees (those who practice devotion). As it is with growing into unconditional and spiritual love, true devotion is usually achieved after experiencing lower forms of devotion. Everyone (even animals) has it to some extent, although it is more developed in some than in others.

1. **Indifferent and superficial.** This is the lowest form of devotion. This type of person has no real desire for devotion, but, when seeing genuine devotion in others, he/she will imitate the behavior, words, and feelings expressed by the real devotees. In this superficial stage, it takes a long time to reach the state of true devotion.

2. **Selfish motivation.** This type of devotion is motivated purely by self-interest. A selfish person has some worldly or religious purpose in mind, and indulges in devotion for an ulterior motive such as wealth, fame, power, and so forth. At first, he/she usually dislikes or disdains real devotees, but gradually changes after his/her selfish motives are fulfilled. He/she will eventually learn to love others and find true devotion by being in the company of true devotees.

3. **Simple and ordinary.** This type of person becomes restless due to the struggle, pain, and suffering he/she sees and experiences in the world. As a result, he/she seeks security and protection from a Higher Power. The lower aspect of this devotion is found in animals, such as a dog's abiding loyalty to its master. Even if the dog's guardian is the poorest of the poor, to the dog he is the king of kings, and nothing can shake his devotion to his master. Such devotion is simple and ordinary, yet contains innocence and purity. Similarly, in people with this type of devotion, such a devotee does not see the faults or weaknesses in the object of his/her devotion. This aspect of worldly devotion eventually develops into a high order and the devotee is freed by a longing to have only the love of God present within him/her.

4. **Logic and reason.** This is a person who wants to know and experience devotion and God, but is thwarted by the reasoning of his/her own mind. Though devoted to knowledge and the finite mind, this type of devotee is conflicted with changing

ideas and doubts. What is gradually learned, however, creates belief and eventually faith in the infinite capacity of Spirit—leading to genuine devotion.

5. **Wisdom.** This is a different type of devotion from the other four types, because such a person, having inner wisdom—superior to outer knowledge—inherently knows of truth and devotion. This type of devotee is wise and intuitive, understands universal principles, and knows the difference between religion and spirituality. When spiritual timing, grace, and opportunity avail themselves, this "old soul" is ready to surrender and give all to devotion of the highest order: service to the Eternal Soul Essence.

What type of devotee are you? Few, if any of us, have perfect devotion, but it may behoove us to reflect on our devotional nature in light of these distinctions. Perhaps we possess and express aspects of all five. Self-awareness in this innate facet of love may assist us in devoting ourselves with grater resonance, heart, and soul.

Service

Only a life lived for others is a life worthwhile.

—Albert Einstein

When we live in loving service to all others, we are at the same time living in loving service to God. We don't focus on or see the personality or ego-self in others; we see through that worldly illusion to the real and True Self. This clarity of inner vision will eventually fulfill our healing journey and our life's purpose.

When you learn to live for others, they will live for you.

—Paramahansa Yogananda

Throughout the ages, the most beloved and influential leaders and kings have known how to truly serve. We're not talking about illusionary, worldly power here, but the power of integrity and wisdom that inspires love and devotion in others. The wise and true masters of life surrender pride and ego to the service of Divine Love.

One of the wonderful rewards of life is that no one can truly help another without helping herself or himself. The gift is given to both the giver and to the receiver. By serving others, we in essence serve ourselves. We often hear the phrase "what goes around, comes around." This may be appropriate not just in the sense of karmic retribution, but also in the joy one feels "coming around" as a result of our acts of giving and serving. Not that that's our only motivation, but, when it feels so good, we want to give more.

> *By serving others, we in essence serve ourselves.*

In the purest service, the one serving and the one being served are one. This is true equality. Some have resistance and difficulty in being of service to others. Others have difficulty in allowing people to serve them. The great George Bernard Shaw said, "Independence? That's middle-class blasphemy. We are all dependent on one another, every soul of us on earth."

By allowing others to serve us, we serve them. By serving others, we are serving ourselves. It is a beautiful cycle of giving and receiving, and a reflection of the sacred interdependence and interconnectedness of life. The miracle in this flowing energy of healing resonance humbles, bonds, and unites us.

In the time we have it is surely our duty
to do all the good we can to all the people we can
in all the ways we can.

—William Barclay

Humility

The practice of service develops humility. When we have humility, we love to serve—we live to serve. One of the most profound examples of love, humility, and service is revealed to us from the New Testament. In the time of Jesus Christ, according to Jewish custom, the host of a dinner who felt honored by the presence of his guests would wash their feet. If, on the other hand, the guests considered themselves honored by the invitation, the host did not wash their feet, presumably indicating his higher social status.

During the Last Supper or Passover Meal, Jesus:

> ...Got up from the supper table, took off his robe, wrapped a towel around his loins (as a servant would do). He poured water into a basin and began to wash the feet of his disciples and to dry them with the towel he had around him....

After washing their feet he put on his robe again and sat down with them. Then he asked: "Do you know what I was doing? You call me 'Master' and 'Lord' and you do well to say this because it is true. And since I, the Lord and Teacher, have washed your feet, you ought to do the same for one another. I have given you an example to follow: do as I have done to you.... If you keep this in mind and put it into practice you will be very happy." (John 13:4, 12–17)

"By this shall all men know that you are my disciples, that you love one another as I have loved you." (John 13:35)

Is it possible for us to model this example of love in this day and age? I don't know—I'd like to think so. In any case, there are great lessons to be learned by this model of humble, loving service. As we learn to open ourselves to the Spirit within, we begin to understand the value of "getting out of the way" and allowing the resonance of Divine Love to heal ourselves and serve others. We become clear and open vessels, conduits, and channels for the purest healing vibrations to flow through us. Upon practicing this method of surrendering the limited power of the finite, individuated, personal self to the unlimited power of the Infinite Whole Self, we will merge and become One with this Divine Loving Spirit. It is then that we can be of the very highest service to ourselves and others.

Do not inflict your will. Just give love.
The soul will take that love and
put it where it can best be used.

—Emmanuel

Summary

Studying the nine core-key healing principles and practicing the associated exercises will greatly accelerate your progress on this exciting and transformational journey. The methodology described will reflect back to you who you really are, and accelerate your understanding of how to effectively use your innate ability for healing.

1. Focused Attention.

2. Prayer/Invocation.

3. Conscious Breathing.

4. Inner Listening.

5. Visualization.

6. Entrainment.

7. Intention.

8. Commitment.

9. Love.

> *We need to embrace and resonate with our innocence and sense of wonder.*

By discovering these core-keys within, you will have the tools available to open the self-imposed "locks" and blocks that may restrict the expansive freedom of your soul. Using these sound healing principles is not an arduous task. Through the practice of these simple methods you can learn to fine-tune your human instrument and experience the joy of voicing your soul, bringing about optimal resonance in body, mind, and spirit.

When venturing into new realms of experience—whether in personal growth, vibrational healing, or spiritual awareness—we may all feel somewhat inexperienced at times. Someone once said, "When you're green, you grow; when you're ripe, you rot." I agree. We need to embrace and resonate with our innocence and sense of wonder, and the nine core keys are the best place to begin. As the great philosopher Kermit the Frog once croaked, "It ain't easy being green." Maybe not, but I'm convinced it's much better than the alternatives—and more fun, too!

(((((18)))))

A Healer's Journey and the
10 Steps to Sound Healing

Till it makes you feel all right
Till you're satisfied with your life
Till you know you live in the Light
Till we get the healing done
Oh, till we get the healing done

—Van Morrison

In the summer of 1993, I experienced an unexpected health crisis. I woke up one morning with a sharp, constant, and excruciating pain in my lower back. No matter what position I shifted to, or how I moved my body, the pain continued relentlessly. I instinctively and regrettably knew the source of my suffering: a kidney stone. I was familiar with the nature and intensity of the pain, because for more than 10 years I suffered from this chronically painful condition, occurring at different times in each of my kidneys.

Previously I was hospitalized on several occasions and injected with painkilling drugs to help alleviate my misery. Over the years, doctors would suggest doing surgery to remove the troublesome stones, but I chose instead to explore natural, alternative remedies—not wanting to be "cut up" unnecessarily.

Although I've subsequently discovered some wonderful alternative healing practices, unfortunately, none of the alternative practitioners I consulted with at that time seemed to agree on a healing regimen for kidney stones. After exploring numerous therapies with little success, I was told by one "natural doctor" that I could get healing results only by spending thousands of dollars on his "unique" therapy and supplements! Another said there was nothing that could be done because the formation of kidney stones was due to genes and was completely hereditary. A highly regarded nutritionist said my problem was due to my being vegetarian. Another said it was best to be vegetarian, but that eating spinach and tomatoes created the oxalate-formed stones. By the time a so-called expert told me kidney stones are created by cooking with aluminum cookware, I was tempted to get stoned!

Thankfully, since that time I've learned much more about kidney stones and the nature of pain, but on with the story. During the 1980s, I was hospitalized on four separate occasions with a painful stone. First in one kidney, then the other, taking turns. Each time—after release from the hospital with no surgery—I succeeded in releasing the stone on my own, but it usually took up to seven or eight painful weeks to do so. And I never fully healed the issue.

Now there I was again, disheartened by having to confront the same painful situation. To make matters worse, I hadn't renewed my health insurance, which had expired two months earlier, so I didn't have the "luxury" of hospitalization or pain-reducing medications. I thought, "What should I do? How can I heal this once and for all?" The pain beckoned.

At the time, I had been working professionally in sound therapy for more than a year and knew which frequencies would support my kidneys. As I was trained in using a therapeutic tone generator, I routinely listened to my sound machine to obtain pain reduction and vibrational support for any stressed body system. However, the pain from the stone in my right kidney was so intense that nothing seemed to relieve it.

"Stone" Therapy

Finally, I decided to meditate and seek inner guidance. I began breathing deeply and diaphragmatically, silently saying my invocation while allowing my body to gradually relax. I then humbly asked Spirit for support and guidance in releasing my pain and in healing myself.

After a few minutes, soft sounds began to come through me. Then louder, more vigorous sounds were released. To my surprise, rhythmic, harmonic, and multiple overtones started flowing from my voice while I simultaneously experienced an array of beautiful color and light-infused visualizations within. I surrendered myself to this vibrational experience and lost all track of time as I felt cleansed and uplifted by the sounds.

From time to time I came out of the meditation state, examined my feelings and experience, and returned again to the sonic meditation process.

I noticed that some of the sounds coming from me felt as if they were extensions of sounds I used to make as an improvisational jazz singer. I remembered that, when singing, I frequently tried to "push the envelope" vocally and felt I needed to express energy and feelings that sometimes couldn't be contained by melody and lyrics. Only certain spontaneous sounds, rhythms, and intonations could fully invoke the yearnings and expressions of my soul.

I felt in that moment of meditation I had expanded the "envelope," or left it completely. I got in touch with something within myself that I subconsciously had always been in search of but never quite reached or found. It seemed to emerge from my voice, in its sound, in the moment.

> *Only certain spontaneous sounds, rhythms, and intonations could fully invoke the yearnings and expressions of my soul.*

After what seemed to be minutes—but was actually three to four hours—my pain was completely gone. I felt intuitively that I had passed the stone from my right kidney and released it from my body. This was confirmed later by X-ray and validated my newly found belief in the healing power of toning and meditation.

I also learned, however, I was not out of the woods yet. The X-ray showed another stone lodged in my left kidney. Because the pain generated by kidney stones is usually caused by their movement out of the kidney and through the urinary tract and bladder, I was unaware of this second stone.

Inspired by my success in releasing the first stone, I felt reasonably confident that I could release the stone from my left kidney. I subsequently toned and meditated daily for several weeks, trusting that I would eventually succeed with the support of Spirit and a commitment to daily practice.

After approximately two months, I felt soreness in my bladder one morning. Though not particularly painful, while urinating I experienced a tingling sensation accompanied by a feeling of release. Again, I intuitively felt that I had released the stone from my left kidney. Upon reviewing the results of a subsequent X-ray, the doctor—to his obvious surprise—found no evidence of a stone in either kidney! I was elated and felt very grateful for my healing experience.

Getting to the Source

I felt further validation in my toning practices and was indeed happy to have experienced such profound healing. However, my new concern was in getting to the source of my health issues.

I knew that I needed to change or heal whatever was causing my kidney stones.

I began by greatly reducing my consumption of "low vibration" foods that weaken the immune system, such as "dead" processed foods, sugar, salt, and carbonated beverages. Already vegetarian, I simply added more "high vibration" natural foods, such as nuts, grains, and fresh, raw, organic fruits and vegetables that raise one's frequency. I also started drinking a lot more filtered water.

As a sound therapist, I had an understanding of how the subtle, high frequencies of thoughts and feelings influence and affect the gross, low frequencies of the physical body. I thus shifted my intention to loving my kidneys rather than fearing and resisting them. I also began a daily toning regimen of projecting the regenerative power of vocal harmonics and overtones into my kidneys.

Over the next several years I experienced only one minor attack of kidney pain, which I released within hours, and I have been completely free of pain and kidney stones ever since. During that period of time I also achieved success in healing and releasing several other health issues, including a colon blockage, chronic knee pain, TMJ, and chronic allergies, which I had experienced for many years.

Perhaps the deepest and most personally valuable healing I experienced is also the most difficult to quantify and articulate because it took place within the subtle, inner regions of the body-mind and stimulated shifts in consciousness. Consequently, I achieved a much greater inner peace, and an appreciation for the various stages of growth and awareness that occurred throughout my healing journey.

Heal Yourself

Don't let anyone tell you what you ought to say,

'Cause maybe you can say it in a better way.

Don't let anyone tell you what you ought to do,

'Cause there's no one who does it quite like you.

So Heal Yourself, get out and join the dance.

Just trust yourself, it's time to take a chance.
And love yourself, you don't have to hide
Heal Yourself, believe in what's inside!
Some people need to learn
what they're always trying to teach.
Some people need to practice
what they always like to preach.
Don't rely on them
or wait for their relief,
Believe in your own dream
and live your own belief!
And, Heal Yourself, finish what you start,
Don't judge yourself, keep following your heart.
Just trust yourself when you've gotta make a choice,
Heal Yourself, listen to your inner voice!
They're pulling on your coat, my friend,
Selling you their points of view
But trying to change the world,
Is not the way for me or you.
We can only change ourselves
If we truly want to heal,
Let's open up our hearts
To live and love and feel!
And heal ourselves, there's just no other way
To have it all, we've got to give it all away.
So, trust yourself, it'll come right back to you
And you'll Heal Yourself, if love is what you do!
Now, love yourself, don't take my word for it,
Just trust yourself, you're gonna get the benefit.
Don't judge yourself, and be afraid to fall,
Heal Yourself, and you can have it all!

—Wayne Perry, *In Chantment*

Vibration Foundation

As a result of my extraordinary sound healing experience I was inspired to make several important changes in my personal life and in my sound therapy practice. In my daily regimen, I committed to loving and supporting myself in a more disciplined manner, with regularity in specifically focused toning exercises and meditation practice. I found that, though it takes a lot of self-discipline to meditate regularly, meditation *develops* self-discipline. And regular meditation creates the strongest foundation possible for personal empowerment and self-actualization, which are vital to healing and sustaining resonant wellness.

In my sound therapy practice I released any remaining dependency on complicated technologies and sound machines, deciding instead to implement a more natural, organic methodology for healing. I simplified my practice to focus on self-empowering techniques such as the use of toning, vocal harmonics, breathwork, and meditation to effect healing from within. I also created brainwave entrainment recordings and healing instruction recordings to support others in easily practicing and learning the principles and exercises I had used during my own healing process.

One of these powerful and important healing exercises (which is included in my four-CD recording series, *The Secrets to Healing with Sound and Toning*) is outlined in the next section—a guide for healing any issues of stress, pain, illness, or disease. When these exercises are understood and practiced, you will be able to change your vibrational frequency, release or transform energetic blockages, and create and maintain body-mind harmony.

The 10 Steps to Sound Healing

Since the human body tends to move in the direction of its expectations—plus or minus—it is important to know that attitudes of confidence and determination are no less a part of the treatment program than medical science and technology.

—Norman Cousins

Earlier we discussed the Three Rs—three types of sound that differentiate various results that can be achieved with their proper use. Here, we'll return to these toning sounds (Relaxing, Releasing, and Regenerating) as a foundation for building a strong and focused healing methodology. With detailed specificity we will expand these basic and important

Three Rs into 10 Rs, which will represent not only associated sounds but also a practice guideline for using the 10 Steps to Sound Healing. When used as a toning and healing exercise, the steps will enable you to specifically change, release, transform, or heal any body-mind health issue that you choose to work with.

At times you may wish to use this exercise for relieving physical discomfort or pain. At other times you may use the process for healing deeply rooted emotional issues or for repatterning old psychological programming. The healing principles are exactly the same. The only components that may shift are your intention about what you want to heal, and where you focus your attention and healing energy in the body. The healing principles remain constant.

1. Clearly and honestly **recognize** the issue you need to heal.

Before you can transform a frequency pattern, you need to recognize its present form. Although a frequency imbalance may crystallize in our bodies as illness, its vibrational roots reach into the emotional, mental, and spiritual levels. The more completely you can consciously know, feel, and experience your true feelings, the better you will be able to transcend them.

> *Before you can transform a frequency pattern, you need to recognize its present form.*

Begin by silently saying the Sound Invocation, or whatever prayer or invocation feels appropriate to your needs. Ask your Higher Self for clarity and guidance in whatever part of your mind-body needs healing in this now-moment.

Listen to both your rational mind, or left brain, and to your feelings of intuition, or right brain, for the answer. Give yourself ample time to be clear about what needs your attention, but be decisive—you can always return to the process later for work on additional issues. Trust yourself. Recognize and identify, very specifically, what you need to change, release, transform, or heal.

Then, without biting off more than you can chew in your first healing session, hold the specific issue—whether physical or emotional—clearly in your mind's eye or awareness. The process of recognition is an essential first step, because only by recognizing the forms your signature frequency has taken is it possible to consciously transform them.

2. Accept **responsibility** for creating this issue for your ultimate highest good.

All of our frequency patterns and health issues are self-created. We may not immediately and consciously understand how and why we are responsible, but being willing to allow for the possibility that we may be responsible opens the way for healing awareness to occur.

In this step, you need to consciously take responsibility for the issue you have identified, because, if you have the ability to create it, you also have the ability to un-create it. Assuming responsibility in this manner empowers you to heal yourself.

Responsibility for healing is taken when you make the conscious choice to change and then act on that choice. When you take action in this way, you realize that responsibility carries no blame and fault, with their associated judgment, guilt, and punishment. Blame implies wrongdoing, and no "wrong" was done when you made a choice that may have been best under the circumstances at the time. In the present, however, that choice may no longer serve you, and may function only to produce disharmony.

One of my clients suffered from chronic fatigue and hypoglycemia, both of which impacted her work and social life. When inquiring about her past history she told me that she received attention as a child only when she was ill or in pain. As she grew older, she learned to manipulate family members into taking care of her by playing a victim role. She perpetuated this behavior into her adult life and relationships. Through sound healing, she was able to discover within herself a deeper intention to experience love and intimacy. She was able to take responsibility for her attitude and behavior, and create a happier life. She also healed her chronic fatigue and hypoglycemia in the process.

In sound healing, responsibility means the ability to understand and accept our participation in our illness, without self-blame or self-judgment. We release the tendency to reactively blame ourselves, others, or God, and realize the importance of being responsive as a form of "response-ability."

Accepting responsibility is an incredibly empowering experience that will lead you into the heart of self-awareness and openness to your healing potential. Opening, trusting, and following your heart will result in a resonant and receptive state necessary in taking the next important step.

3. Openly **receive** what this issue offers you.

Before we can give something away, we must first receive it. For example, the love that we receive teaches us how to give love to others. If we openly receive love from family and friends, we are likely to give freely of our love to others. If we have been shown and given anger, shame, and blame, we may display and give out the same. This is also true for what we give ourselves.

In order to give ourselves, or anyone else, healing sound or vibrational energy, we must first be open and able to receive it. This also means we must be able to receive—without fear or resistance—the stress, pain, and disease that comes into our lives. This does not mean we have to hold these conditions in our bodies. On the contrary, we need only allow ourselves to be fearlessly present as an open conduit through which these disharmonious frequencies may pass through to be released and transformed. Remember the principles behind the Noise Pollution Exercise. Again, what we resist, persists.

What stresses and disables the body most is when we close ourselves off from our life experiences, resisting change and growth. When we allow ourselves to trust and receive life in each moment, we automatically become free from the deleterious effects of stress that are generated from outer circumstances. We move toward peace, gratitude, resonance, and oneness within ourselves.

Man can only receive what he sees himself receiving.

—Florence Scovel Shinn

The Gifts

Another very important part of the reception process lies in our ability to receive the lesson and gift that is contained within every problem, pain, illness, or disease. This is described simply and beautifully by author Richard Bach in his book *Illusions*: "There is no such thing as a problem without a gift for you in its hands. You seek problems because you need their gifts." As we open ourselves to receive these gifts, we find an abundance of blessings and support awaits us.

This process also involves a willingness to acknowledge and open the feminine energy that exists within your signature frequency—whatever your gender. It is inherent in the female principle to open and receive. By using this principle appropriately, you prepare yourself to better access and use the male principle of "release." As you continue to receive, integrate, and balance these two polarities within your signature frequency, you will deepen your receptivity and capacity for creating wholeness.

During this third step to healing, you may wish to begin toning soft, relaxing sounds corresponding to feelings of receiving.

4. Allow thankfulness to enter your heart by returning to a state of loving trust and re-appreciation.

A thankful heart is not only the greatest virtue,
but the parent of all other virtues.

—Cicero

What is the most natural and appropriate response to receiving a gift? Hopefully, appreciation. As we learn to receive and appreciate the lessons and gifts contained in our pain or health issues, we defuse the charge of fear and resistance around the issue. When we can feel gratitude for our discomforting and threatening situation, we can better understand and accept the purpose in it. We can affirm that this condition has given us something; we have received and appreciated it; this issue has served its purpose and may now be released.

I frame this step as re-appreciation because it infers that we were, at one time, in a state of appreciation. In other words, perhaps the issue in need of healing at some point shifted our attitude of appreciation to one of fear or resistance. Or our feelings and attitude may have contributed to our healing issue and somehow nullified our appreciation.

Whether this is the case or not, the important point here is to allow yourself to embrace, feel, and express your appreciation for what has been received and learned from your health issue. Upon fully experiencing gratitude and appreciation, you can now expand into healing resonance. During this fourth step to healing, you may wish to begin or continue toning soft, relaxing sounds corresponding to feelings of appreciation.

Love is to resonance, as fear is to resistance.

5. Fully and completely resonate with your issue without holding any resistance in your body-mind.

There are many ways in which we can view and use the phenomenon of resonance on our healing journey. Through resonance, vibrational harmony can be re-established, returning the body to its natural state of wellness. Love is to resonance, as fear is to resistance. Love fuels resonance. Fear fuels resistance.

Joy and wellness always involve love and resonance.
Pain and disease always involve fear and resistance.

—Wayne Perry

Resistance

The resistance to the unpleasant situation is the root of suffering.

—Ram Dass and Paul Gorman

Change is one of the issues most resisted, but change persists and is constant. Once we inhabit a state of resonance, resistance to change is minimal. Resistance—whether conscious or unconscious—causes us to view our bodies, relationships, and life circumstances from the perspective of being at the *effect* of outer conditions rather than seeing ourselves at the *cause* of our condition. Before we can fully move into resonance, we must go to this source in our awareness so that we may gain clarity in identifying areas of resistance within us and take responsibility for them.

> *The antidote for fear is love. The result of love is resonance.*

Because we can be terribly hard on ourselves at times, it's important to look at our issues of fear and resistance without self-judgment and condemnation. We need to totally accept ourselves as we are, and the most complete form of this acceptance is love. So the best way to come into resonance with ourselves is to love ourselves just as we are.

The antidote for fear is love. The result of love is resonance. Choosing and affirming self-love and resonance within ourselves establishes a frequency of thought that can permeate our entire vibrational body. We can then recognize and assess areas of fear and resistance within ourselves and simply change the frequency by consciously choosing resonance.

New Paradigm

The old approach to healing was to isolate, attack, and destroy illness or disease. The new paradigm in healing is to integrate, restore, and harmonize the whole. This holistic perspective assists us in seeing new ways in which we can align, balance, and tune the body-mind, enabling it to heal itself and prevent disease.

When we can view disease, such as cancer, as a living part of ourselves that needs love and resonance to heal—rather than as a vehicle of death and destruction—we can experience our Wholeness. When we can release our fears of death and disease, and learn to trust in our capacity to love, resonate, and heal ourselves, we will know our Oneness.

> *The new paradigm in healing is to integrate, restore, and harmonize the whole.*

This attitude of resonance engenders trust, peace, and gratitude, which create a sound environment for healing, transformation, and harmony. Our thoughts and beliefs are responsible for the feelings and emotions we experience. In turn, these feelings give birth to our physical experiences and perceptions. Integrating these parts of ourselves by practicing loving frequencies of thought will resonate us into the heart of wellness.

It is essential to the sound healing process that you tone relaxing sounds—gradually increasing in volume—throughout the Resonance Steps. (Refer to Chapter 8 and Chapter 16 for additional details.)

The Resonance Exercise

The following steps will assist you in achieving the optimal resonance during your process.

≈ Visualize a form that represents your health issue, pain, or illness.

≈ Imagine a sound that represents and reflects the nature of your pain or illness.

≈ Listen to, and softly tone, the sound of the pain or illness.

≈ Breathe deeply into the form and sound of the issue while feeling your connection to it without fear or judgment.

≈ Using all your senses and awareness, resonate with your condition for as long as it takes until you feel resonance and oneness within yourself.

≈ Upon achieving resonance, affirm that your issue has served its purpose and is now no longer needed, and then gradually increase the volume and intensity of your toning in preparation for release.

≈

6. **Release** the issue.

We have now arrived at the point of release. After recognition of your issue, accepting responsibility for it, openly receiving the lessons offered, feeling renewed appreciation, and fully coming into resonance with it, you can now release it.

If offered the opportunity, most of us would probably prefer to take the quickest, easiest, shortest, and cheapest way possible to effectively heal ourselves. Well, guess what? This is it! However, don't be fooled by a popular misconception that you can immediately switch from Recognition (Step #1) to Release (Step #6), and be successful in fully releasing your issue. This is the tendency of those who are impatient and inexperienced in self-healing. As you patiently and methodically approach each healing step as an opportunity to achieve deeper self-awareness and transformation, you will find your efforts well rewarded.

Volume

One of the most vital components of the Release step is the proper use of vocal volume during toning. In order to successfully raise the frequency necessary to facilitate an effective release, we must raise our toning volume sufficiently. It is also important, however, to not overextend or strain the voice.

To find an appropriate volume level, imagine yourself in a somewhat noisy environment calling out to a friend to get his/her attention. Or, calling to someone from a distance of a hundred feet or so. You wouldn't scream at the top of your lungs, as in a warning of danger. This level of volume, with repetition, could potentially damage your vocal cords.

You would, however, amplify your volume by raising your pitch and focusing the sound of your voice. This illustrates an approximate volume level for toning release work. Along with regular toning practice, allowing your feelings and intuition to guide you will also assist in achieving the best volume needed at any given time.

Cleansing Sound

Release sounds rely mostly on volume, vowels, and breath to effect the "frequency cleansing" necessary for releasing blockages, pain, and vibrational toxicity from the body. The vowels fully open the sound of the voice. Conscious expulsions of breath, while simultaneously toning vowels, will facilitate the release of unhealthy or dissonant frequencies.

Affirm that your health issue has served its purpose, is no longer needed, and is now ready to be released. While holding this clear intention in consciousness, tone the sound of the issue—creatively, intuitively, and uninhibitedly. Allow your body to move, as needed, to better facilitate release. You may stand, sit, or lie down, whatever best supports your process. Continue for as long as needed to effect release. Be patient.

As you feel a sense of complete release, "peak" your vocal volume while simultaneously visualizing a burst of white light within you. Or, you may experience the issue releasing and merging into a beautiful violet flame. Be creative; the importance lies in clearly feeling, seeing, and sounding the release of your issue. Lovingly bless and release the disharmonious energy into the Source of sound, light, and love, to be transmuted to a higher frequency.

Depending on the depth of the issue and the clarity of your intention, the time needed to effect a release may vary between mere moments to many minutes during any given healing session. According to your nature and needs, you may chip away at an issue over several weeks of short sessions. Or, you may find it more conducive to deeply focus for 30 minutes or more in one or two intense release sessions. Be flexible, and use both common sense and intuition to guide you. You are now ready to move to the next step in the healing process.

7. Allow your whole body to **relax.**

After experiencing the inner-cleansing power of the release process, it is important to give the body-mind ample time to relax and be calmed. There is no fixed time for this healing step, as needs will vary according to the individual.

The Relaxing Breath Exercise

One of the best vibrational tools always available to us is our breath. The following steps describe in detail the Relaxing Breath technique.

- ≈ Close your eyes and exhale completely.
- ≈ Calmly and diaphragmatically breathe in and out through your nose.
- ≈ Breathe in gently and deeply for three counts or seconds.
- ≈ Hold it for a moment, then breathe out for six counts.
- ≈ Do this three or four times and notice how you feel.
- ≈ You should feel sufficiently relaxed now, but continue longer if necessary.

≈

Consciously breathing in this manner is one of the most effective ways to quickly induce relaxation.

Relaxing Sounds

The use of relaxing sounds will deepen and sustain your relaxation. If you're not already toning relaxing sounds, begin doing so now. Allow gentle vowel sounds or humming to flow through you, calming and soothing your whole being. Feel the sound vibrations flowing throughout your whole body, relaxing each and every body system. Feel your heart, lungs, and chest relax. Feel the relaxing energy expand, permeating your solar plexus, abdomen, and chakras. Feel it calming and relaxing your arms and legs, hands and feet, fingers and toes, throat, face, and head.

Continue toning in this manner until your whole body, mind, and feelings are completely relaxed. Stay alert and awake, however, as you are now ready to access the most powerful healing step.

8. **Regenerate**, renew, and restore body-mind harmony.

Some healing modalities may be successful in releasing a health issue, but may not be as effective in preventing its return. With sound healing we address this important distinction.

If you want to permanently release an issue—pain, illness, tumor, disease, addiction, whatever—you need to go to the source and regenerate the body-mind at that vibrational level. You need to tune or change the frequency of the condition so that it does not return. Of what benefit is it to release a health issue and then find it reappearing weeks, months, or years later, to plague you once again?

After we release something, what are we left with? What do we now have? If we ponder this question carefully, we find that we are left with nothing—a space or void. If we ignore or fail to "refill" the space, it is possible that what we have released will return. Could this be why cancer goes into remission, only to resurface later? Or why those who have released severe pain, lost excessive weight, or kicked an addiction find their efforts in vain when the problem reemerges? Let's explore this further.

> *To fully follow through with your healing, you need to fill the space left by your release.*

Filling the Void

To fully follow through with your healing in this step, you need to first fill the space or void left by your release. Then, by using the Core Key Healing Principles along with regenerative sound, you can "re-form" the vibrations that were "un-formed." This process will enable you to rebuild and regenerate the energetic source of your issue and tune your signature frequency.

The Regeneration Exercise

The following exercise will assist you in "filling the void" and permanently healing your health issue.

≈ Create a clear intention to heal and regenerate yourself.

≈ With your eyes closed, bring a deep breath in—as if coming through the crown of your head—and send your out-breath into the void created by your release.

≈ Imagine your breath as a healing white light nourishing and filling the void within you.

≈ Simultaneously with each out-breath, begin toning vowel sounds, allowing them to blossom into sonic bouquets of overtones and vocal harmonics. Project them into the space or void within you.

≈ Get your mind out of the way and allow your Soul-Self—through intuition—to guide your tones, pitch, sounds, and imagery.

≈ See the space or void slowly begin to fill and take a new form, exhibiting all healthy functions and characteristics.

≈ Affirm that the new vibrational pattern created is a permanently higher frequency, transcending and replacing any old disharmonious patterns.

Note: If your healing issue is of a physical nature, visualize vibrant, healthy cells and tissues, resonating perfectly and harmonically in that organ or body system. If your issue is of a subtle-energy nature, such as emotional, visualize white light, harmonic colors, or any outward symbol that represents to you Wholeness and transformation. It is also important to embrace a feeling of unconditional love for yourself during the regeneration process. Sound, light, and love function as harmonics connecting you to the natural resonance of a healthy state. These higher frequencies can prevent old, released vibrational patterns from reconfiguring.

Higher frequencies can prevent old, released vibrational patterns from reconfiguring.

≈

Follow-Through

Our healing process should be comprehensive and thorough for optimal effectiveness. An essential part of this process is a matter of follow-through. In sports, a golfer, baseball batter, or football kicker must use a proper follow-through in his swing or kick—after making impact with the ball—for optimal accuracy and maximum distance. Similarly, in martial arts the best defensive maneuver when being attacked is not to resist the impact of the strike or kick, but to redirect the force of the blow using its momentum of follow-through to protect ourselves and avoid potential harm. This is the same principle at work, seen from a different perspective. It also reminds us of the appropriateness and importance of resonance over resistance.

Whether in sports, martial arts, or the healing arts, understanding the energetic principle of follow-through is essential for achieving success. Likewise, the principle of regeneration is necessary in moving us successfully from releasing disharmonious energy to healing and transforming it, thus enabling us to "follow through" to our two remaining healing steps.

9. Feel gratitude for your healing experience by re-acknowledging its source.

As in Healing Step #4, the act of re-acknowledgment infers that we were at one time in a state of gratitude and thankfulness. At this point in the process, however, your acknowledgment and appreciation are not directed toward the gift or lesson in your health issue. The purpose of this step is twofold. First, to gratefully re-acknowledge benevolent Spirit, the Divine Loving Consciousness, as the True Source and Real Facilitator of all healing. And second, to acknowledge yourself for "response-ably" having the courage, commitment, and humility to make the effort to heal yourself, which is indeed the purest form of self-love.

During this healing step, it is important to cease any toning and quietly listen to the silence or the Inner Overtone. Remain in this receptive, meditative state as long as desired and convenient.

10. Rejoice in your Wholeness.

The final step of this healing practice is to simply allow yourself to fully feel, experience, and express the joy in your Wholeness. To rejoice is to celebrate your return to joy. To enjoy, or be "in joy," greatly assists in accessing and expressing your natural resonance without the tendency to take yourself too seriously. It lightens any heaviness, allowing the Spirit to soar!

> *Freely rejoice in the love of your soul, and the soul of your love.*

Joy is the source of delight and bliss. Love is the source of joy. And in our highest and purest reality, only love is real. Freely rejoice in the love of your soul, and the soul of your love.

The most appropriate toning and healing sounds to best support this last step are any sounds that reflect and correspond to feelings of joy. Resound and rejoice.

≈

It has been my intention in this chapter to facilitate a clear understanding of the 10 Steps to Sound Healing by delineating the various healing principles, therapeutic techniques, and toning practices. Keep in mind, however, that there may be gray areas and overlapping principles involved with their best application. A comprehensive and effective healing practice should never be rigid or inflexible. Your personal experience, creativity, and intention, ultimately, should always reign.

For example, you may notice some regenerative overtones coming through your voice while toning release sounds, you may need to tone additional relaxing sounds after the regeneration step, or you may find yourself unexpectedly toning release sounds during any of the steps. Trust yourself. Trust in sound. Resonate with your feelings and instincts. Use these sound healing steps as foundational guidelines to support your freedom and ability to heal yourself.

The 10 Rs or Steps to Sound Healing

1. **Recognize.**
   Toning sound: Relaxing or silence.
   Primary frequency: Mental.

2. **Responsibility.**
   Toning sound: Relaxing or silence.
   Primary frequency: Mental.

3. **Receive.**
   Toning sound: Relaxing.
   Primary frequencies: Emotional/Mental.

4. **Re-appreciate.**
   Toning sound: Relaxing.
   Primary frequencies: Emotional/Mental.

5. **Resonate.**
   Toning sound: Relaxing, gradually moving to Releasing.
   Primary frequencies: Physical/Emotional/Mental.

6. **Release.**
   Toning sound: Releasing.
   Primary frequencies: Physical/Emotional/Mental.

7. **Relax.**
   Toning sound: Relaxing.
   Primary frequencies: Physical/Emotional/Mental.

8. **Regenerate.**
   Toning sound: Regenerative.
   Primary frequencies: Physical/Emotional/Mental/Spiritual.

9. **Re-acknowledge.**
   Toning sound: Silence.
   Primary frequencies: Physical/Emotional/Mental/Spiritual.

10. **Rejoice.**
   Toning sound: Any joyous sounds!
   Primary frequencies: Physical/Emotional/Mental/Spiritual.

The Three Toning Sounds

1. **Relaxing Sounds.**
   Calm, soothe, comfort, and prepare the body.

2. **Releasing Sounds.**
   Cleanse, free, unburden, and relieve the body.

3. **Regenerative Sounds.**
   Restore, rebuild, renew, reform, and heal the body.

(((((19)))))

The Sound Healing Sanctuary

We continually create and manifest our own reality and our perception of it.

—Wayne Perry

A useful and adaptable format in which you may maximize your effectiveness with the 10 Steps to Sound Healing—or most any toning exercise—is the Sound Healing Sanctuary. It is a sonic meditation and fundamental process that incorporates guided imagery, along with toning and sound healing principles. The purpose of the Sound Healing Sanctuary is to create the optimal atmosphere and inner environment for practicing and developing powerfully personal sound healing experiences.

Whenever I receive reports from someone having difficulty achieving the desired results from his/her sound healing, upon researching the situation, I usually discover his/her struggle is due to one or more of the following reasons:

≈ Failure to fully understand or implement the Core Keys/ Healing Principles.

≈ Insufficient time or application given to the 10 Steps to Sound Healing.

≈ Lack of self-confidence and/or discipline.

≈ Withholding love from oneself and others due to a lack of forgiveness.

The first three may be improved with increased awareness, time, practice, and the meditative focus offered by The Sound Healing Sanctuary. For the maximum benefits, however, the last issue, forgiveness, may need to be addressed in more detail.

Forgiveness

Those who can't forget are worse off than those who can't remember.

—Anonymous

Forgiveness is all-powerful.
Forgiveness heals all ills.

—Catherine Ponder

One of the key issues that can impede one's success in creating wellness with sound is the inability to forgive. A lack of forgiveness is resistance. Forgiveness is resonance. If the will remains in resistance, it stays dependent on that which it is resisting. For this reason, in the forthcoming detailed description for creating and using your own Sound Healing Sanctuary, we will focus on a powerful forgiveness exercise. However, you can also adapt and use your Sanctuary for gaining deeper access to healing any other issues.

> *Forgiveness is resonance.*

The Sound Healing Sanctuary Exercise

(You may wish to read aloud and record the following exercise and instructions. You can then repeat this closed-eye process, as needed, for enhancing your healing experience. The Healing Sanctuary is also available on compact disc as part of my *Healing with Sound and Toning* instructional series.)

Begin your healing inner journey by closing your eyes, and breathing deeply and diaphragmatically. Allow your body to relax more and more with each exhalation. Invoke and evoke the Divine Spirit within, using the Sound Invocation or a prayer of your choosing. Open your heart and feel your body being filled with sound, light, and love. Imagine your soul-essence being activated and rising up and out through the crown of your head. As it rises further, look down from your soul-consciousness and see your physical body below, sitting peacefully. Continuing to rise upward, passing through the ceiling or any other obstructions, your soul now soars up and out into the sky above.

While playfully riding the breezes and dancing on clouds, start to visualize the ideal location for your Sound Healing Sanctuary. In search of the perfect environment, you creatively ponder all your choices: a majestic mountaintop, a beautiful valley, a lush forest, a desert island—there are no limits to your imagination. Perhaps the perfect place is under the sea where you can breathe underwater, or in a subterranean cavern deep within the bowels of the earth. Maybe it exists on a cloud—or even another planet! Anywhere and anything is possible.

Once your intuition has guided you to the ideal pristine location, identify all the details in your environment. Notice any particular objects that contribute to the healing beauty of the space: flowers, bushes, trees, grass, rocks, streams, ponds, waterfalls, butterflies, birds, rainbows—anything that contributes to the beauty and resonance of the surroundings. The more specific you are, the easier your visualizations will become and enhance the exercise.

Now, imagine the ideal structure for your actual Sanctuary. Start with the type of building or house you've always wanted to live in. Perhaps it's an ancient, regal-looking castle or a sprawling estate. Maybe it's a modest country cottage, a log cabin in the woods, or a simple thatched hut on an island. Again, be creative; let your visions unfold. Perhaps you see an ultra-modern steel and glass structure, a wild and unusually designed house, a geodesic dome, a hidden cave in a mountainside or underground, or even an underwater "bubble house." You are the visionary architect and intuitive designer!

Once you've clarified the structural details of your Healing Sanctuary, see yourself standing at the door or entryway. Feel the joyful anticipation of exploring your own unique healing space. Now, see yourself entering and immediately feeling a sense of peaceful security as you stand inside. As you scan the inner environs, notice that there is a room designed to meet your every need: a room for research and study, another for creative expression, a room in which to confer with the experts and masters on any subject, a play room, and rooms for eating as a king or queen, entertaining, exercising, relaxing, sleeping, meditating, and much more. Pay attention to all the details: space, floors, rugs, walls, artwork, windows, design, lighting, colors, shapes, sizes, and so forth. Manifest and create whatever you want. Everything you could ever need exists within your *Healing Sanctuary*.

Now, find your healing room. As you are intuitively guided through your Sanctuary to this special healing chamber, once again, you feel an enhanced sense of anticipation. As you approach the doorway, you find yourself slowly entering a moderately large, round room. Feeling as though you are walking on a cloud, you glide toward a comfy chair on a small platform in the center of the room. You mount the chair and, while settling into it comfortably, feel as though it was custom made for you. Relaxing into this sacred space, you are now ready for the healing process.

(At this point, you will consider and realize what Divine purpose is there for you in the moment. You may work with any sound healing principle or exercise, including name toning, chakra balancing, Tantra Toning, sacred sounding, resistance, or release work. For example, if your inner guidance is to work with releasing a particular physical or emotional issue, hold an intention to follow the 10 Steps to Sound Healing and their associated toning sounds. However, because the failure of many healing modalities is often rooted in holding onto judgments and a lack of forgiveness, we will now address healing this issue.)

≈

With full clarity of intention and commitment, perform each step in the following three exercises.

Forgiveness Exercise #1

Close your eyes and recall a situation when you said or did something that hurt another's feelings. Or, perhaps it was something you didn't say or do that you should have. Recall the other person's actions and responses. Think about what you did or didn't say or do. Examine why you behaved as you did. Re-feel your feelings from that time, and notice how you feel about them now. Be willing to take full responsibility for your behavior.

Now, bring before you the image of the person you hurt or offended. Look deep into his/her eyes and ask for his/her forgiveness. As you hold his/her gaze, say, "I'm sorry for what I said and did. It was thoughtless and inconsiderate. Will you please forgive me?" Or, "My behavior was thoughtless, rude, and insensitive. Can you ever forgive me?" Speak from your heart and mean it.

Imagine the person responding back to you: "It's okay. I understand. I had completely forgotten about it. I forgive you. I forgive and release you." While sustaining eye contact, allow yourself to fully receive his/her forgiveness. Feel the release in your heart and body as you are freed from this past experience. Gently tone an "AH" release sound from deep within you to complete the closure. Sincerely thank the person who has forgiven you, and release him/her. Feel the joy that comes when the truth and the love is found and expressed.

Allow another person from whom you need forgiveness to come before you. Repeat the same process with this individual, until the energy is cleared between both of you. Continue by calling in any person from your past that may need to receive your apology, and from whom you need forgiveness. Strive to achieve closure with each and every individual. Upon feeling complete with this process, move on to the second exercise.

≈

Forgiveness Exercise #2

This exercise involves your forgiveness of others. Recall a time and situation in which someone hurt your feelings. Perhaps it was a friend or family member who said or did something that deeply hurt you. Or someone who neglected to say or do something you feel he/she should have. Recall the person's words and actions. Do you think his/her behavior was intentional, or just thoughtless? In what ways did you react? How did you contribute to the conflict? Did you hold the pain of the situation in your heart? Re-feel

> *Experience within yourself the peace and freedom of increased resonance.*

your feelings from that time and notice how you feel about him/her now. Are you willing to take full responsibility for your part in this situation?

When you feel ready, invite the person that hurt you into your Healing Sanctuary. See him/her standing before you and look deep into his/her eyes. Now imagine that he/she is apologizing to you and asking for your forgiveness. See and feel his/her sincerity. Hear him/her say to you, "I'm sorry for what I said and did. It was thoughtless and insensitive. Can you ever forgive me?" Or, "I'm sorry for being so thoughtless and inconsiderate of your feelings. It wasn't my intention to hurt you. Please forgive me." Listen to and receive his/her humble apology. If any resistance comes up and you have difficulty in accepting the apology or offering him/her your forgiveness, remember how it felt when you asked another for forgiveness.

When you are able to, accept his/her apology and offer your forgiveness by saying: "It's okay. I know you didn't mean to hurt me. I forgive you." Or, "I'm sure you meant no harm. I'm happy to forgive you and release you." Say this with complete honesty and sincerity while sustaining eye contact. Allow yourself to fully release him/her from your mind, heart, and body. Gently tone an "AH" sound from your heart—releasing the past, while opening to the healing available in the present moment. Experience within yourself the peace and freedom of increased resonance. Feel the joy that comes when truth and love is found and expressed.

The weak can never forgive.
Forgiveness is the attribute of the strong.

—Mahatma Gandhi

Allow another person in need of your forgiveness to come before you. Repeat the same process with this individual until the energy is cleared between both of you. Continue by calling in any person from your past who hurt you in any way and needs your forgiveness and release. Hold an intention to achieve healing and closure with every individual in your life, living or dead, past or present, as needed.

Note: If there is someone in your life whom you have a difficult time forgiving, particularly if it is a parent, the following technique may be helpful: When this person is standing before you and making eye contact, imagine him/her appearing younger and younger. For example, see him/her as he/she might have looked in his/her 20s. Notice his/her youth, innocence, gestures, and expressions. Empathize with his/her lack of knowledge, confidence, and experience, and his/her fears and insecurities. Then see him/her as a teenager—even more confused and lacking in understanding. Chuckle at his/her peculiar-looking clothes and appearance. Now see him/her as an endearing little 5-year-old just needing love and attention. Sympathize with

> *I forgive you, I accept you, I trust you, and I love you—even when I don't understand you.*

this child and imagine how he/she might have grown insensitive to others because of the way he/she was treated. Embrace him/her and offer your nurturing, acceptance, love, and understanding. Reassure and forgive him/her. Finally, see this child smile and run off, giggling with youthful joyousness, and departing—along with any feelings of pain and enmity that you may be holding. Allow these feelings to be replaced by compassion, harmony, and peace.

≈

Forgiveness is the answer to the child's dream of a miracle by which what is broken is made whole again, what is soiled is again made clean.

—Dag Hammarskjold

This completes the second step in the forgiveness process. When ready, you may move to the third and final step, which is the most important, for it involves forgiving yourself. And, we can't offer total and lasting forgiveness to others, or fully receive it, if we haven't forgiven ourselves.

Forgiveness Exercise #3

Recall a time and situation in your life when you may have sabotaged yourself, or made a severe error in judgment. Think about the details of the situation and the various thoughts and feelings you had at the time. What were your actions? In what ways did you judge yourself and "beat yourself up"? Are you holding within yourself any feelings of inadequacy, blame, or self-doubt? Identify the self-destructive thoughts and feelings you wish to forgive and release.

When you feel ready, see the image of yourself entering your Healing Sanctuary. This image of you may be at any age—childhood, adolescence, adulthood, or present. Welcome this part of yourself to appear before you. Look deeply into your own eyes and feel your connection to, and acceptance of, this part of you. Listen intently as this image of you says, "I'm truly sorry if I hurt you and let you down. I meant you no pain or harm. I was not thinking clearly or acting wisely, but I will try harder. Please forgive me."

While sustaining eye contact with this image of yourself, draw him/her to you. Embrace and hold him/her gently and whisper into his/her ear, "It's all right. I forgive you. It's not important. Let it go. It's over. I forgive you. I love you." Now repeat the following intention and affirmation: "[Your name], I forgive you, I accept you, I trust you, and I love you— even when I don't understand you." (Repeat three times.) And finally, "I forgive you, I accept you, I trust you, and I love you—*especially* when I don't understand you!" Together with your "harmonic self," tone a long "AHHH" sound from your heart, along with any other tones and sounds that may need to be expressed.

Close this step of the exercise by giving the image of yourself a hug and a kiss on the cheek. Tell him/her that you will always be there for him/her, and lovingly release him/her into the Light. Feel the joy that comes when the truth and the love is found and expressed. This completes the third and final step of the "forgiveness process."

(If for any reason you feel incomplete in your forgiveness, you may need to lengthen the duration or repeat some portion(s) of the exercise.)

≈

Returning Home

Take an opportunity to give thanks to the Divine Spirit within for the gift of healing forgiveness. After a few moments of silent gratitude and meditation, you may now prepare to leave your Sound Healing Sanctuary and return home. Remember that you can return to your Sanctuary any time you wish to do deep toning and healing. Practicing your sound healing exercises in the solace and sanctity offered within your Healing Sanctuary can be an extraordinary tool for assisting you in discovering and tuning your signature frequency. Through this sonic meditation process, you will learn to concentrate your vocal healing energy and accelerate your journey to Wholeness.

You may now exit your Healing Sanctuary with a celebratory burst of "vocal vibration" that magically uplifts you through the ceiling and roof, and up into the sky above. Feel the breezes caress and support your spirit as you begin your journey back to where you started. Your spirit soars through the air, joyously returning to the place from where you first departed. Seeing the structure below, you float gently down through the roof, hovering in the room while observing your sacred body temple waiting patiently below. You slowly lower yourself, finally merging back into your body.

Upon feeling fully present in your body, take a deep breath and ground yourself by toning a long, descending vowel sound. While doing this, expel all the oxygen from your lungs, and bring your attention down to the base of your spine. Slowly open your eyes, take a fresh breath, and stretch your body—as you feel invigorated and joyous, yet calm, relaxed, peaceful, healed, and enlightened. Welcome home!

≈

(((((20)))))

Secrets for Sound Healers

We transmit to others that which we most need to receive.

—Wayne Perry

When Mike arrived at my office for his first sound healing session, he complained of having a severe headache that day and a bronchial infection for four or five weeks that he couldn't shake. After a brief consultation, I conducted a diagnostic voice analysis to determine Mike's stressed body frequencies and then moved on to the sound healing.

Mike lay down on my healing table, and I explained to him the nature of the vocal sounds that I would be using, and generally what to expect. After toning Mike's needed frequencies into various areas of his body, including the cranium, spinal column, meridians, and certain chakras and energy points, we completed the healing session. The whole process took about 45 minutes.

Upon arising from the healing table, Mike exclaimed that he felt quite energized, yet relaxed and refreshed (a common response), and that his headache was completely gone. Before he left my office, I suggested that he drink plenty of water to assist his body in releasing toxins, and we scheduled another session for him the following week so that I might teach him some toning and self-healing techniques and exercises.

Mike called me in two days and excitedly shared with me that his bronchitis seemed to be gone, and he was really looking forward to this next session. I was happy to hear that he had such rapid and dramatic results, as it is difficult to predict the outcome of a healing treatment because we "co-created" the experience, and also because everyone has their own unique signature frequency.

When Mike came in for his next session, I taught him some key exercises for using his voice to do release work and other self-healing sounding. He then asked if we could do another sound healing session. Because we hadn't planned one, and his bronchial infection seemed to have healed,

I asked Mike why he felt the need for another healing. He replied by telling me a fascinating tale of recent events in his life.

When he first came to see me, Mike said that he hadn't been completely honest with me. The day before he scheduled the appointment had been what he described as the worst day of his life. In addition to being informed of recent developments that might require him to sell or close his business, Mike also learned that his father was seriously ill. To make matters worse, on the same day, Mike received the results of medical tests that indicated he had an abdominal tumor that was malignant. Feeling overwhelmed by the day's tragic news, he went home to compose himself and meditate.

Upon finishing his meditation, Mike said that he got up and did something he had never done after meditating: He turned on the television. Normally, he said, he feels the need to sustain the peace and quiet after meditation, but this time he felt a need to see "something" on the TV. The first thing that appeared on the screen was me performing a sound healing demonstration on a female subject. Mike said he stood transfixed, watching the unusual experience. He felt intuitively that he could derive benefit from this unique healing modality and called me the next day to schedule an appointment.

Feeling both saddened and intrigued by his interesting story, I asked Mike why he hadn't shared these details with me on his first visit. He said that, without having any knowledge or experience with sound therapy, he wasn't convinced that it could help with his cancerous tumor. But he felt it probably couldn't hurt either, so he decided a trial run with his bronchitis might be appropriate and insightful for him. And now that he felt more confidence in the sound healing process and comfortable with me, he was anxious to move forward in exploring sound and toning in the hopes of helping his more serious condition.

I felt fine with this, as I know each individual is unique in the unfolding of his/her awareness and healing. Some need to study research, books, and other resources to satisfy their doubts or left-brain needs. Others naturally trust their gut feelings or intuition, and still others use a combination of both sides of the brain to arrive at a trust level necessary to properly participate in a healing modality.

I expressed to Mike that, although a sound healing session may certainly help him, he shouldn't hold any expectations about the outcome, and that it was important to also follow his doctor's advice in supporting his medical needs. Mike said that he understood and wanted to proceed with the session.

A Sound Healing

During the sound healing treatment I focused my vocal harmonics and overtoning directly into the area of the body where Mike's tumor was located, toning his weakest frequencies while still allowing the sound to guide me intuitively, as well. This is initially a vocal-vibrational-scanning process. Upon feeling connected to his energy frequencies, my intention was to assist him in releasing the detrimental frequencies responsible for the dissonance/malignancy in his body, then energizing and supporting the resonant and healthy cells. I also first suggested to Mike that he allow himself to express any release sounds, if it felt natural and comfortable for him to do so, at any time throughout the process.

After almost an hour, we completed our second sound healing session, with Mike enthusiastically sharing that it felt "miraculous." Explaining that he could feel a warm and intense pulsing of energy flowing throughout his body, he was simultaneously having various light-infused visions while a blissful cleansing was taking place. "Miraculous, truly miraculous," he kept repeating. Now, I know I'm no miracle worker, but often, the unique vibrationally energetic experience that occurs during a sound healing—when one is open and receptive—can indeed be quite dramatic.

I suggested to Mike that he listen daily to toning recordings of his deficient frequencies that I provided him with, practice the toning exercises I taught him, and continue to meditate and ask for inner guidance and support. These efforts would deepen and extend his healing experience until our next session. I also invited him to attend our ongoing toning circle and sound support group that I host for sound and toning practitioners. Mike replied that he was anxious to do his toning and sounding, and would love to attend our next group.

The Good News

At the second toning group he attended, Mike announced that he had something important to share. He first asked if it was all right with me if he could briefly describe his initial experiences of discovering my work, and how we were working with sound and toning to support the treatment of his cancerous condition. I assured him that it was fine with me, after which he gave us an update.

Mike said it had been five weeks since he had received the medical tests informing him of the malignant tumor, and that on this morning he had just received the second set of test results. To his doctor's amazement,

Mike's tumor had shrunk from the approximate size of a golf ball to the size of his little fingernail! The doctor said he had never seen such rapid improvement in such a short period of time, and he gave Mike 90 percent hope for recovery.

Because Mike had earlier agreed to follow his doctor's recommendation to undergo radiation treatments, the doctor automatically assumed that Mike's dramatic improvement was a direct result of this therapy. And perhaps it was. Although he was hesitant to express it to his doctor, Mike was totally convinced that his sound therapy sessions were responsible for his much-improved condition.

A Question of Healing

Whatever circumstances contributed most to Mike's healing—his attitude and clarity of intention, listening to needed sounds, toning exercises, sound healing sessions, or radiation therapy—his experience points to some frequently asked questions:

≈ If more than one healing modality is being used, as is often the case with those in catastrophic health crises, how can we determine which modality is the most effective?

≈ Can we validate or quantify a healing experience?

≈ Is it possible to isolate or separate the efficacy of the healing modality from the healer?

These are valid and intriguing questions, but do the answers lie in further research, double-blind studies, and left-brain analysis? Do we rely on personal experience or gut feelings and intuition? Are these questions even answerable?

The study of the "new physics" suggests that many of our old concepts and standards for judging so-called reality may be skewed and antiquated, as we learn more about quantum mechanics and the real nature of matter, time and space, light and sound frequencies, human consciousness, and healing. Perhaps a more useful question might be: If a healing modality appears to be working and giving me value, and there is no risk of danger to anyone involved, shouldn't I have the freedom to take personal responsibility to explore and use it, if I so choose?

In the spirit of this question, let us proceed in exploring in more detail the potential benefits of using the vibrationally complex—and virtually untapped—healing resources contained within the human voice.

The Healing Power of the Voice

Every pitch that is a natural pitch of the voice will be a source of a person's own healing as well as that of others when he sings a note of that pitch.

—Hazrat Inayat Khan

Although it continues to be studied and analyzed, no one knows exactly the full healing potential of the voice. Perhaps its power lies in the fact that, unlike the limited technology of sound machines and tone generators, the voice is connected to and is an expression of the limitless, Infinite Loving Spirit within, and can literally voice your soul. No matter how advanced our technology becomes, a machine will never have a soul.

In 1981, French bioenergeticist and sound-worker Fabian Maman was involved in experiments that studied the effects of various sounds on the nucleus and electromagnetic fields of human cells. After introducing an assortment of acoustic musical instruments, he observed that the most impressive results occurred when he toned or sang musical scales into the cells with his unaccompanied voice. Maman states in his book *The Role of Music in the Twenty-first Century*, "It appeared that the cancer cells were not able to support a progressive accumulation of vibratory frequencies.... The structure disorganized extremely quickly. The human voice carries something in its vibration that makes it more powerful than any musical instrument: consciousness...."

Healing Others

Similar to how we may focus and direct our vocal toning sounds into any of our body systems for our own healing, we may also use the same principles and techniques in assisting others in their healing. Being a sound healer for others—whether professionally, or in support of friends and family—involves a great commitment to be of service.

While presenting sound healing methodologies in seminars at various conferences in this country and abroad, I've been inspired and delighted over the years by the passionate interest expressed from those exploring this growing field. In addition to desiring personal healing and transformation, more often than not, those drawn to this important healing modality wish to be of service to others, as well. It is for this reason that I feel compelled to elaborate further on some of the principles and techniques discussed in earlier chapters—with regard to healing with the voice—in context of the role of a sound healer.

The Methodology

When studying the therapeutic possibilities inherent in the voice, it's helpful to begin by examining the voice's unique sounding capabilities and their relationship with regenerative sound. Although no singing or musical experience is necessary for the development of your vocal instrument's innate healing power, its proper use with regard to vibrational principles will greatly enhance your effectiveness in using your voice as a healing tool.

> *Raising your vocal pitch can tune that energy center, or assist in its better functioning.*

There are four principle components that will enhance and expand the vibrational healing capacity of your voice. Any of these four methods may be used individually. However, a thorough understanding of all of them, along with their appropriate integration and use, will give you mastership of the "healing voice."

1. **Body-Mind Sound Correlations.**

   The use of specific sounds, vowels, pitches, and notes can assist you in vibrationally supporting areas of need in one's signature frequency. For example, a particular vowel sound can assist you in opening or clearing a blocked chakra, meridian, or other energy center of the body. Raising your vocal pitch can tune that energy center, or assist in its better functioning. The use of specific musical notes can support particular body systems and their functions.

   There are several effective means for identifying the most appropriate and supportive toning sounds. As discussed earlier, some of these methods include voice analysis, vocal scanning, applied kinesiology, dowsing, or just fine-tuning your intuition. Once these specific sounds, pitches, or notes are determined, they may be toned directly into any particular area or body system as needed.

   Additional benefits may be achieved by using toning sounds in various combinations or "mantra-like" patterns for restoring vibrational balance, achieving brainwave entrainment, and supporting the body's overall cellular function. These vocal sounds may also be recorded and replayed for ongoing use as desired.

2. **Vocal Harmonics and Overtoning.**

   As you develop the technique of using your voice to create vocal harmonics and overtones, you will gradually concentrate the regenerative power of your sounds. This is in part due to the creation of multiple tones and note frequencies, which in turn create multiple waveforms and more concentrated energy. You may use these energetic multiple frequencies to target specific areas of the body that need support, regeneration, and vibrational healing.

The more you practice overtoning, the more confident and effective you will become in mastering the many dimensions of sound that you can create with your voice. Learning this "magical methodology" will reward you with one of the most powerful healing tools for naturally achieving and sustaining wellness. (To review these techniques, refer to Chapter 11 and Chapter 12.)

> *Learning this "magical methodology" will reward you with one of the most powerful healing tools.*

3. **Encoding Sound.**

To increase the effectiveness of healing with the voice, it is important to understand that you may "encode" vocal sounds to be carrier waves of intention. When a clear intent is focused into and through the sounds you are toning, it empowers those sounds by encoding them with a specific healing intention. As discussed in earlier chapters regarding regenerative sound, this encoding process can concentrate the vibrational healing energy of the vocal frequencies produced.

But this is only half of the encoding process. The other half has to do with your consciousness while producing vocal sounds. For example, if you are harboring negative thoughts or emotions toward anyone—including yourself—while trying to hold a healing intention, you will not be successful. Irrespective of your intention, your overall level of consciousness, capacity for love, and signature frequency is automatically imprinted and encoded into every sound that you make, and has an effect on you, and on whomever or whatever you project sound into.

> *You can only heal yourself or others to the extent that you can love yourself.*

This "sound effect" may be subtle or dramatic, depending on various factors, including the amount of space between you and the object or one receiving the sound, the duration of time elapsed during the sounding, your focus and mood, the receptivity of the object or one receiving, and environmental conditions.

The essential thing to remember is that love and the soul are inextricably linked to your intention when creating potentially healing vocal sounds. And you can only heal yourself or others to the extent that you can love yourself. So, loving yourself is the first and most important step in being effective in encoding sound as a carrier wave for healing with the voice.

4. **Sacred Sounding/Spiritual Healing.**

In spiritual healing with sound it is necessary to set aside your logic, reason, left brain, and personality-ego-self, so as to allow your voice to be a sonic conduit through which your soul may express itself. By this "sacred sounding" of your spiritual essence, you are able to deepen your vibrational connection with the Divine Source. The intimate connection with your higher self is both an act of self-love and an opportunity for profound healing to manifest from within.

Non-calculative, spontaneous, sacred sounding can hold extraordinary benefits because the state of your outer body is always precipitated by your inner state. In this manner, as you experience your oneness with the Inner Overtone you will be a receptor for sacred sound and be able to transmit this unifying vibration to others.

> *This process will lead you to mastery of the healing voice and the voice of your soul.*

By holding this intention and releasing the need to control the process and results, your trust in your soul, sound, and self will build and strengthen. With this sound spiritual practice, your vocal sounds will literally guide you through the appropriate tones, pitches, and body systems in need of resonance. Eventually, this process will lead you to mastery of the healing voice and the voice of your soul.

Because all healing is really self-healing, when you choose to heal and serve others you are merely a facilitator in supporting another's transformation process. You become a conduit, a catalyst, and co-creator of healing energy in loving support of another, and this is a sacred relationship and responsibility. To honor this special relationship and facilitate the optimal healing experience and sound environment, it is important to understand the key elements in the sound healing process.

Unlike working only on ourselves, when facilitating healing for others, there are additional dimensions to the process, which enable the subject or client to feel at ease and to actively participate if he or she chooses.

Other elements will deepen and enrich your "vibrational palate of harmonics." I briefly touched on some of these points earlier when describing Mike's initial experiences with toning and sound healing. Let us now examine more fully the key ingredients and steps for facilitating healing for others.

> *When you choose to heal and serve others you are merely a facilitator in supporting another's transformation process.*

Seven Steps for Sound Healers

1. Assist in putting the healing subject at ease by generally explaining what he or she can expect during the sound healing session. For instance, the sound of vocal overtoning may seem very strange and "otherworldly" to one who has never heard these types of harmonics before. I've known the sounds to fascinate some, yet frighten others.

   It is also a good idea to tell your subjects how long the session will last; share a few points on what you will and won't be doing, and invite them to participate in any ways that are appropriate to the process and comfortable for them. For example, I always explain to my clients that I will be making some "strange" sounds, and not to be alarmed; there may be some gentle touching, but nothing of an intimate nature. I usually invite them to close their eyes, breathe deeply and diaphragmatically during the process, and tone along with me if at any time they are inclined to express a sound (although most are a bit inhibited to do so).

   In short, establish a good bond and an open, communicative resonance with your subjects to help them feel comfortable with the uniqueness of the process. This will assist them in being receptive to the vibrational benefits of the healing. If you are working in a professional context, you should always inform clients that the sound healing session is not a substitute for any needed medical treatment, and that if they have health issues they should consult their doctor.

2. Always ask your subjects' permission to enter their "personal space" before beginning the sounding process. Most of us get a little uncomfortable when someone is within close proximity to our bodies and focusing their attention on us, particularly if they are not a close friend or family member.

Upon receiving their permission, try a few test tones while in this close range. The reason for this is that oftentimes, even though your subjects have given you permission, they are trying to be receptive but are still inwardly resistant or nervous. As you become more experienced with the process, your sensitivity will develop in being aware of any resistance in your subjects. You can help turn this momentary blockage into resonance by acknowledging them with understanding and patience.

The vocal toning and healing process may often require that you tone directly into a specific area of the subjects' body, such as the cranium, spinal column, or a particular chakra center. To concentrate the energetic effect of the vibrational frequencies, it is often beneficial to at times cup your hands around your mouth (as if you are shouting to someone far away) and press them gently on the subjects' body while toning the sound into that area.

If you explain in advance that there will be no painful, sexual, or inappropriate touching involved with this method of sound-healing-resonation, most will feel comfortable with the process, and usually enjoy it. Although this may be somewhat similar to "hands-on healing" methods, some sound healers refrain from any kind of touching altogether. Use your common sense and intuition, and do what works best for you and your clients.

3. Before beginning the sound healing process, be sure to clear your personal energy by saying a prayer or invocation to the Divine Loving Spirit to allow harmony and protection to be present for the highest good of all concerned. Then ask for permission and support in using your voice, body-mind, and soul as a loving instrument of service for facilitating resonance and healing.

This invocation must come from your heart, not your head. Although it is usually said silently within, if you feel comfortable saying it aloud, and it would put your subject more at ease, do so. Invite them to say it with you, if it feels appropriate. Be flexible and in the moment. As mentioned earlier, the important issue here is getting out of the way, and being an open conduit through which vibrational healing energy may naturally flow. (Refer to Chapter 16.)

> *Release any expectations regarding the outcome.*

4. Start with a clear intention about your subjects' needs, what you want to accomplish, and how you can best be of service. Then release any expectations regarding the outcome.

   Know that with this attitude and intention everything will unfold perfectly, irrespective of any conscious or unconscious projections and expectations that you or your subjects may hold. By always remaining in the present moment you allow yourself to be guided and empowered by Loving Spirit.

5. Allow yourself to be intuitively and vibrationally guided by the sounds coming through you. During the healing process, sensitize yourself to the resonance of your vocal sounds by listening to them, feeling them, and allowing the sounds to spontaneously lead you through whatever harmonics, tones, pitches, and notes might be needed. You may begin by toning specific vowels, but gradually, as it feels appropriate, let the sounds themselves direct you.

   It can also be helpful to let the sounds and your intuition guide you to various body systems and areas that may be in the most need of resonance. Learn to trust in sound. As mentioned earlier, it can yield wondrous rewards and benefits.

   > *You can't predict or control the "magic" of healing.*

   Another issue to consider is the amount of time needed to conduct a proper healing session. This is an area in which your intuition, aided by your sounds, may assist you in knowing exactly when enough is enough. The time may vary greatly. At times, energy blockages and frequency excesses may be balanced or released in mere minutes; other times, it could take hours. Healing issues frequently need to be "chipped away at" and returned to from time to time, and may require additional sessions.

   I've often experienced cases in which clients' healing occurred before the session started, or after they left my office. You can't predict or control the "magic" of healing. Once there is a sincere intention to heal and receptivity is created, healing can occur. Again, be open, flexible, and trust in yourself and the sound healing process.

6. Upon completing the toning and sounding portion of the healing session, allow for a period of "sacred silence" and quiet meditation to facilitate the full absorption and integration of all healing vibrations and frequencies. This is a time for the body-mind to relax, reflect, and regenerate in a sort of "sonic afterglow."

At times you may have subjects who will journey deep into their consciousness (or sometimes, unconsciousness!) and need extra time to come back to their body-awareness. In a patient manner, give yourself and your subjects ample time to gradually make the transition from the inner to outer body. It's important that by the end of this step, both of you are fully present and grounded.

If it is not too loud or jarring to your subject, gently striking a bell or a drum at the end of the meditation may assist in the grounding and signal to them the close of the session.

7. Offer sincere and heartfelt thanks to Loving Spirit for all blessings and support of the sound healing experience. A grateful heart resonates the most fully.

Upon giving thanks, ask for support in clearing your energy field of any remaining "vibrational residue" that might impede your optimal resonance. When working on or with others in healing work, it is easy to take on or absorb your subjects' energy, which may be unhealthy for you. You may better effect this clearing process by the release of short expulsions of breath, burps, and other sounds. Allow your intuition to guide you spontaneously through completion of this process. Usually one or two minutes of clearing is sufficient, and you will feel refreshed. Finish with another grateful acknowledgment of Spirit.

≈

To better facilitate the co-creation of wellness when being of service to others in their healing, sometimes all that may be needed is for us to listen. There is no sure way that we can fully know all the underlying circumstances behind others' pain, imbalance, or disease. They may not know this themselves. There may be further growth, lessons, or karma that they must experience before releasing or healing an issue. At times, all we may be able to offer them is nonjudgmental support, an open ear, and love—trusting that healing occurs at the perfect moment.

The Healer's Role

If all healing is self-healing, why would one need to seek out a sound healer?

We may not need to, if we feel knowledgeable and confident enough to use sound appropriately in our own behalf. If, however, we can gain knowledge or benefit from another healer, why not? If we want to learn to be adept at law, medicine, politics, or plumbing, it would benefit us to study with an expert in those fields. Healing is no different.

Healing is not curing. Curing belongs to the realm of doctors, drugs, and disease. Healing has more to do with taking responsibility for one's physical, emotional, mental, and spiritual health. And health belongs to everyone. The role of a sound therapist, a healer, or even a sound machine is simply to act as a "jumper cable" to assist us in healing ourselves. A good healer recognizes this distinction and knows when to be assertive, and when to get out of the way, thus supporting the client in creating a healing experience.

> *After working with a healer, one should always feel nurtured, hopeful, better informed, and empowered.*

Sometimes, just being present with a receptive vibration or as a sounding board is all that is needed to support an individual in his or her healing process. Keep in mind, also, that it may not always be readily apparent if one has an unconscious attachment to some part of his or her illness or imbalance, thereby preventing its release. Timing can indeed be everything. A good healer knows this and never forces an issue. And most importantly, during or after working with a healer to co-create wellness, one should never feel shamed, intimidated, confused, or dis-empowered; one should always feel nurtured, hopeful, better informed, and empowered.

By realizing the healing potentials available to us and within us, we can maximize our healing results. At times, it may be most beneficial to seek out the expertise of another whose knowledge and experience may assist in jump starting some part of us that feels blocked or stuck. At other times, we may find more benefit by developing and using our own innate healing power.

Each one of us, however, is both a transmitter and a receiver. We are all social and interactive beings by nature, so there is much to be gained by sharing and being open to our capacities to both give and receive vibrational energy and the healing power of love—sometimes as the healer, other times as the "healee." Trusting in the clarity of our intention and the use of our intuition will always direct us toward the role that holds the most value for us at any given time.

Indeed, all it may ultimately take to heal our signature frequencies is loving ourselves enough to be willing to stay in the present moment—and keeping in mind, and heart, that the healing love we offer others will always be proportionate to the healing love we offer ourselves.

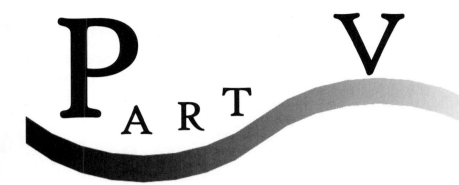

The Inner Voice: The Way In Is the Way Out

*On the supreme Sound Current of the Word
we descended into the human form, and by
that same current we shall ascend to our
primal Source.*

(((((21)))))

Being of Sound Mind

*The greatest discovery of my generation is that man can
alter his life simply by altering his attitude of mind.*

—William James

When the finite mind surrenders to love, the infinite soul wins.

—Wayne Perry

Except for the soul, the mind vibrates at the highest frequency in the body. Whereas the soul expresses itself through the infinite vibrations of sound, light, and love, the mind operates through the finite vibrations of sensing, thinking, and reasoning. The soul lovingly imbues us with a positive resonance and a spirited affinity for holistic connection with each other, a natural Oneness. However, the mind—due to the ego—is inherently negative and fears for its own survival because it sees all others as separate from itself.

From a worldly standpoint, the mind is a phenomenal instrument. It can solve problems, allowing us to make tremendous advances in our quality of life. The mind has developed technology to not only make life easier, but also enable us to save lives. The mind generates our facility to learn and communicate more comprehensively through language, education, and the arts.

From a spiritual standpoint, however, the mind is finite and limited. The greatest mystics and masters tell us that the soul, or "real self," is dominated by the mind, and the mind is dominated by the senses. In turn, the senses of the body are ruled by the objects of sense. The soul is covered and surrounded by mind and matter. Though we are a combination of soul, mind, and matter, in present manifestation we are mostly matter, meagerly mind, and imperceptibly soul. Our state can be thought of in the same way as metal covered by rust and then by mud. In this state the metal does not behave as metal and is not attracted by a magnet. Its association with the mind taints the sensitivity and purity of the infinite soul.

Spiritual masters also say that, because the mind and soul are inextricably "knotted together" at the eye center in the forehead of the body, this presents a dilemma for the total expression and liberation of the soul. But by shifting the polarity and focus of the mind's attention within, we can gradually wash away the debris of mind and matter, thus enabling the soul to follow its natural attraction to the Sound Current—the Inner Overtone.

> *For the soul to gain freedom from the delusions of the mind, the soul must ultimately access the inner Sound.*

In order for the soul to gain freedom from the delusions of the mind, know its infinite nature, and return to its true Home, the soul must ultimately access the inner Sound. The body-mind, too, will fully experience the therapeutic benefits of overtoning, vibrational healing, and true spiritual awareness once it knows the bliss of hearing this Sacred Sound and Celestial Melody within. But until this "momentous merging" occurs, the tendency of the mind is to fight and resist its transformation and ultimate destiny.

As the moon is bright due to the light of the sun, so the mind is bright due to the light of the soul—the brightness depending on the amount of the light received. The inherent nature of the mind is materialistic, outward and negative. When it faces outwardly it is associated with matter, and when it faces inwardly it gets illumination from the soul.

—Maharaj Sawan Singh

Spiritual Gems

> *We must develop physical and emotional self-control, vigilant mental discipline, and regular spiritual practice.*

If we wish to achieve real self-mastery and liberation of the soul, we must develop physical and emotional self-control, vigilant mental discipline, and regular spiritual practice. With this discernment and self-discipline, the mind can then control the senses and the soul can control the mind. By this self-empowering process, we return the soul to its rightful place of dominance so that we can be truly free.

The Nature of the Mind

*A man who is "of sound mind" is one who keeps the inner
madman under lock and key.*

—Paul Valery

Your automobile may be an efficient instrument for travel, but it
must be guided and kept under control. Having no will of its own, it
needs your will. If you allow your car to drive itself, just think of the
damage it can do. It cannot think or see; it can be driven properly only
by your trained guidance.

Exactly the same situation exists with your mind. The mind can be an
excellent servant, but makes a very poor master. As your servant, it can
be of great benefit; as your master, it may wreak havoc upon you. Fire
also is a good servant, but the moment it is out of control, it becomes
destructive. It may light your way in the darkness, or it may burn down
your house. Generally, the more useful and powerful an instrument is
when properly controlled, the more destructive it is when out of control.
This is the case with the mind. As the most powerful instrument available
to the soul, it must be appropriately directed. There are practically no
limits to what the mind can do when properly awakened, trained, and
empowered by Spirit.

Until we achieve this, however, our ability to know ourselves, the real
"soul self," is inhibited by the mind's dominant authority. Similar to a
bucking bronco, only with proper taming, training, and guidance will the
rebellious mind surrender and be our friend. So, before we can indeed
know this soul-self, we need to identify and understand the layers between
what the mind thinks and what the soul knows. Then, with the development of the soul's consciousness, we will surely know that we know.

Tuning In

For another perspective of our situation, imagine that you are living
in a time before the advent and popularity of television and movies. The
main source for entertainment was the radio. On Saturday nights, families would gather together and listen to their favorite radio program. Everyone usually had a good time unless the program was affected by the one
thing that could spoil their enjoyment: an interruption of the radio signal
caused by a power failure or, more frequently, by static. The intruding
sound of static could greatly impede a radio's proper transmission.

Similarly, we could view the body-mind in much the same way as a radio. The current of electricity could be seen as the Sound Current that gives and sustains life. We tune our dial and receiver (personal frequency) to pick up the transmission (focused attention) of the station's broadcast (pure consciousness) and adjust the volume (level of reception and expression). Any static (impediment to spiritual awareness) that may occur is the result of scattered attention or misuse due to faulty thought processes.

The happiness of your life depends upon the quality of your thoughts.

—Marcus Aurelius

For a better understanding of this analogy, the thought process can be divided into four "frequencies of static" or categories of "ego-driven thinking":

1. **Fear-based thinking.**

    Occupied with thoughts of anxiety, worry, doubt, confusion, discontent, despair, shame, guilt, regret, resentment, anger, revenge, denial, and so forth, the mind is concerned with what will be or what has been.

2. **Unfocused thinking.**

    Occupied with daydreaming, fantasizing, and illusion, the mind is concerned with what should be.

3. **Interactive thinking.**

    Occupied with thoughts of jealousy, envy, mimicry, vanity, self-image, and how others perceive us, the mind is concerned with what others are thinking about what we are thinking.

4. **Calculative thinking.**

    Occupied with thoughts of power, competition, winning, strategizing, scheming, cleverness, control, defensiveness, manipulation—and often, anger, blame, sarcasm, cynicism, oppression, and deceit—the mind is concerned with how to get it, use it, own it and keep it.

    This fourth aberration of the mind is the most insidious and difficult to overcome, because it is the most commonly accepted, and frequently revered, by society. We are greatly encouraged to be clever, calculative, and competitive, as the only way to survive in this world—let alone be successful.

But there is another way, a way that encourages self-respect, unity, harmony, and honors the Oneness that resonates within us all. It is the natural, Spirit-powered way of the soul. This "way" involves transferring the reigns of rulership of our lives from the calculative and imperfect designs of the mind to the loving and inner-knowing capacity of the soul, thus returning the soul to its true seat of power.

Intellect, Logic, and Reason

Instinct guides the animal better than the man.
In the animal it is pure, in man it is led astray
by his reason and intelligence.

—Denis Diderot

Pure logic is the ruin of the spirit.

—Antoine de Saint-Exupery

All our reasoning ends in surrender to feeling.

—Blaise Pascal

Although the mind may have the useful and appealing qualities of a fine intellect, sharp reasoning ability, and vast creative power, from a spiritual perspective it is our nemesis. Important as it is to know the true soul-self, equally vital is knowing the enemy: the mind, with all of its strengths and weaknesses. This enables us to conquer its wayward and addictive tendencies, so that we may gain the necessary dominion over it.

The mind's primary functions and strengths include sensing, reasoning, logic, intellect, and creativity. These facets of the mind can be invaluable to us when used in the proper context. For example, in creating a foundation for the purpose of analysis, there can be no better instrument than the intellect. Through its logic and reasoning capabilities, the intellect can be very useful for gathering and organizing information, processing data, and problem-solving. Yet when the reasoning function is applied to the decision-making process, frequently the more we reason, the more doubts we create in the mind. The more we think about a problem, the more confused we become. The mind becomes crowded with so much information and

> *We are drowning in information, thirsting for knowledge, and starving for wisdom.*

so many alternatives that lack of certainty and confusion are inevitable. We are drowning in information, thirsting for knowledge, and starving for wisdom.

Objectivity may be the essence of intelligence, and universal love the essence of wisdom. However, you can be loving without being wise, but you can't be truly wise without being loving.

Left and Right Brain

Another difficulty that is encountered when trying to observe and understand the mind is how to achieve this knowledge. Is the intellect an adequate instrument for knowing itself?

One of the major weaknesses of the intellect is its inability to fully understand metaphysics and spirituality because it views them through a lens framed by time and space. And because the intellect processes information through logical thinking, reasoning, and analysis, the mind subjectively shades every perception with its own previous experiences. Most of the activities of our lives are guided by the knowledge generated by this left-brain part of the mind.

The intellect is severely limited in the arena of spiritual understanding because the mind is finite by its very nature. It functions only within the realm of beginnings and endings, cause and effect, and time and space. Attempting to use the left brain to understand spiritual principles and infinite truths is akin to trying to hold the ocean in a teacup! Therefore, the best contributions that intellect can make to the process of acquiring knowledge are to know and observe its limitations.

> *Attempting to use the left brain to understand spiritual principles, is akin to trying to hold the ocean in a teacup!*

We need to spend time regularly in activities that feed our souls and develop our right-brain attributes of creativity, spontaneity, intuition, innocence, trust, faith, joy, and love. Activities such as writing, painting, singing, dancing, toning, and meditating bring our left-brain and right-brain hemispheres into balance. This enhances our life potentials for optimal health, happiness, abundance, and fulfillment with a strong, whole-brain foundation.

The Paralysis of Analysis

Intellectuals may not like or accept it, but the intellect is actually destructive in nature. Whenever you bring the mind and intellect into use, they immediately dissect and analyze an issue. The intellect is the function of the mind—and the power in human awareness—to break experiences into parts. It isolates pieces of information for the purpose of analysis and seeing parts of the whole. It cannot objectively see and experience the whole. This characteristic of the intellect to analyze through reasoning—by breaking things into parts and pieces—is what is responsible for the creation of all our feelings of fear, doubt, uncertainty, and separation.

The soul, however, functions not by breaking experiences apart, but by joining them together by synthesis—with love. By the power of love we experience the wonder and beauty of the whole. When we experience the oneness of the whole we finally begin to see its intricate perfection. To see and experience the "whole of life," we must use other functions of human consciousness.

Some other faculty than the intellect is necessary for the apprehension of reality.

—Henri Bergson

Beyond Time and Space

What exactly are these "other functions of human consciousness," and how do we use them? Whether conscious of them or not, we use them every day. They are intuition, sound, light, and love. All may lead to spiritual experiences because, by their very nature, they transcend time and space.

For example, think of a time when you had an intuition about something. Now try to recall the moment when that feeling came to you. Can you pinpoint the exact minute you felt it? Was it 9:45 a.m.? Or 1:20 p.m.? Can you locate in time precisely when you had that intuitive feeling? Where did this intuition come from? Once we begin analyzing the situation by reflecting on the time frame or source of the information, we immediately leave the receptive and intuitive state, and enter the more limited arena of analysis. The flash of intuition we experience is rooted beyond time and space, in the dimension of Spirit. In the pure intuitive process, no errors are ever made and no time is taken to know the answer. The finite mind can only function within the dimensions of time and space, and cannot quite wrap itself around this "timeless" experience.

Let's explore another example by observing the nature of sound and light. Think of a time when listening to a wonderful piece of music or viewing a beautiful piece of art, when you felt touched or moved by the aural or visual beauty. Try to recall the very instant you felt moved by feelings of upliftment or beauty. Again, can you pinpoint the exact moment in time that you experienced those feelings? The primary sound and light within music and art, respectively, are also spiritually rooted beyond time and space. As soon as we bring in the intellect to examine our feelings, we lose the timeless joy of the experience.

And finally, let us look at the wondrous experience of love. Can you recall the precise moment when your heart became filled with the joy of love? Can you identify the very minute that you first felt the bliss of love?

> *The infinite, transformational power of real love transcends the boundaries of time and space.*

Do you know, as surely as you live and breathe, exactly when an overwhelming feeling of love filled your whole being? The limitless nature and experience of love is, again, beyond the mind's comprehension. The infinite, transformational power of real love transcends the boundaries of time and space—freeing us to ascend to the spiritual realms in which it is rooted.

Love is the greatest of all mysteries. It can be lived, but cannot be intellectually known. It can be experienced, but cannot be understood. It transcends all logic and reason, space, and time. Love is the highest possible experience attainable in human consciousness.

As you can see, we have all had some of these experiences that transport us beyond the limitations of time and space. They move us from the pragmatic left brain to the creative and intuitive right brain. When we are receptive to them, these spontaneous, inner experiences stimulate spiritual awareness—profound "a-has" that bring us to the threshold of the infinite nature of our soul. Many of these experiences are beyond our control and may involve destiny, karma, or the Grace of Spirit. But there are also those inner experiences that are well within our reach by implementing vibrational principles and spiritual disciplines, thus bringing us ever closer to our Eternal Home.

Faith is a higher faculty than reason.

—Bailey

Special Note: Throughout this chapter and the next, I frequently mention the soul going or returning to its True or Eternal Home, Spiritual or

Infinite Source. A clarification must be made here. When considering ascension in consciousness beyond the finite mind to the realms of Infinite Spirit, it's important to remember that—spiritually—there is no time or space. In order for space to exist, there must also be time. Time and space do not exist on the level of pure Spirit, so actually, we are already Home. There is no place to go to in space, and no waiting in time. There is no past; there is no future. There are no past or future lives or events. From a spiritual standpoint, everything is going on simultaneously and we are already One.

> *From a spiritual standpoint, everything is going on simultaneously and we are already One.*

The catch is that we may not have the conscious awareness of our Oneness, divinity, and Infinite Beingness. If this is the case, it may behoove us to go within and discover these truths for ourselves. It's ALL inside.

The Power of Intuition

Intuition…appears to be the extrasensory perception of reality.

—Dr. Alexis Carrel

Intuition is given only to him who has undergone long preparation to receive it.

—Louis Pasteur

Through the instrument of the mind, the soul creates. In fact, looking at Creation from a metaphysical standpoint, Spirit created the whole Universe through the frequency of Universal Mind. We then experience this magnificent creation through the collective consciousness. And it is through the higher creative mind—guided by love and intuition, the nature of the soul—that we access the Sound Current and ultimately return to our Infinite Source.

However, the tendency of the lower mind—the sensing and reasoning components used by the intellect—is to ensnare the infinite soul in the realm of time, space, and causation.

Analysis kills intuition.

The means to transcend the limitations of sensory input, reasoning, and intellect is through intuition, because intuition leads us to real love and awareness. The intuitive faculty is the bridge between the higher mind and the consciousness of the soul. Author and lecturer Shakti Gawain says, "By learning to contact, listen to, and act on our intuition, we can directly connect to the higher power of the universe and allow it to become our guiding force."

Intuition draws upon the total conscious and subconscious experience that lies within the awareness of the individual. In *Anatomy of Consciousness,* East Indian philosopher and author, Ishwar Chandra Puri writes:

> The intuitive process is based upon the entire scope of the individual's experience and knowledge. Not only of one's self (of one's personal past), but that of the whole history of mankind as well! This huge storehouse of knowledge, containing the unconscious memories of the entire experience of human evolution (stored in the "sanskaras," or the soul's accumulated impressions), is accessible through the use of the intuitive process. Intuition is based on this knowledge of the totality of the human experience. By having access to the entire history of human experience, it is easy for intuition (the soul of man) to arrive at the smallest details of a given situation and determine, with absolute precision, everything connected with it.

In the same way that we exercise a muscle group in the body that we wish to strengthen, with regular practice and development of the intuition, it becomes stronger and more trustworthy. In truth, our intuition is never wrong; what is faulty is only our ability to clearly hear it and listen. We are often distracted and confused by dissonant frequencies, such as fearful thoughts and feelings of doubt.

> *It is the intuitive faculty that is the bridge between the higher mind and the consciousness of the soul.*

With mental discipline, emotional self-control, and intuition, we can significantly transform our awareness and harmonize all our personal frequencies. When we fail to trust in our inner knowing, we fall back on fear-based thoughts and calculative thinking. The use of our intuitive faculties is vital to our spiritual growth as it shifts us from vibrations of fear to vibrations of love.

Fear

At its basic root essence, the soul is ruled by love. The mind, on the other hand, is ruled by fear. This is why, in social, political, or religious dogma, fear is so often used to threaten and manipulate the masses. It can work only to the extent that we live in the darkness of a closed mind and the spiritual immaturity of reactive emotions. In this type of environment, we may be prone to various fears, such as fear of not fitting in with society, fear of government oppression, or fear of the "wrath of God."

Power does not corrupt. Fear corrupts,
perhaps the fear of a loss of power.

—John Steinbeck

When we live from our soul, however, we do not allow ourselves to be affected by these types of threats; we are not run by fear. We are moved and ruled only by faith and love.

An open heart and mind, trust in our intuition, and regular spiritual practice are all we need to shift the polarity of our consciousness from a fear-based to a love-based perspective. This commitment to the soul-self then moves us from a painful mind-based struggle, to a joyous soul-based method for living freely.

Spiritual masters say this fear fuels the propensity of the mind toward anger, lust, greed, excessive attachments, pride, and ego. All pain, conflict, doubt, despair, and duality are rooted in some combination or derivation of these destructive and dissonant frequencies. In the same way that a raging forest fire destroys all in its wake, these passions, when allowed to run wild, take possession of the mind and control of the spirit.

Until we achieve mastery over the mind, it will continually run outward for its fulfillment, and we will be overpowered and immobilized by fear. With discipline and infusions of love and faith from the soul, however, the mind will gradually gain trust and surrender to its infinite destiny.

The Ego

The roots of all our fear-based frequencies lie in the primary agent of the mind: the ego, and its limited, self-involved perspective. The mind cannot be purified and controlled until the ego is subdued. Although with great discipline and resolve we may learn to overcome anger, lust, greed, and the bonds of worldly attachments, our egos may still be filled with pride.

My favorite parable on this topic involves a powerful and wealthy king and his life-changing experience with the 13th-century mystic, Kabir, a master of the Sound Current, who was often called the weaver saint.

One day a king was overcome with desire for God-realization and began seeking the company of sages and masters. However, he lived in such luxury that he always slept on a deep mattress of fragrant flowers. One night, when he was going to bed, he heard a noise above him and, on investigation, saw two men roaming about on the palace roof.

"What are you doing here?" he demanded.

"Sir, we are camel drivers and are searching for our lost camels," they replied.

Amazed at their stupidity, the king said scornfully, "How could you ever expect to find camels on the top of a palace?"

"In the same way that you are trying to realize God in your bed of flowers," was the reply.

This greatly shocked the king and completely changed his way of thinking. He abandoned his throne and started to meet with the saints and sages in his own kingdom, but without satisfaction. He then went to India and, after making a thorough search, was still unsuccessful until he reached Kashi. While there, he learned of a wise mystic by the name of Kabir.

After finding Kabir, he asked the weaver saint to accept him as his disciple. "There is nothing in common between a king and a poor weaver like myself," Kabir humbly replied, "and two such different persons could hardly get on together."

But the king pleaded with him, "I did not come to your door as a king, but as a beggar," he said. "I beg of you to kindly give me the gift for which I am seeking." Kabir's kindhearted wife, Mai Loi, also asked her husband to accept him, and the master finally gave in to the king's request.

In a weaver's house, what could the king do other than assist the weaver with menial tasks? Six years passed by, and the king did his work without a murmur. One day Mai Loi entreated Kabir, saying, "This king has now been with us for six long years, he has been eating what we offer him, and has been doing what we order him to do, without uttering a word of complaint. After all of this, he now appears to be highly evolved and deserving, so please give him something."

"As far as I can see, the king's mind is not yet crystal clear," Kabir told his wife.

Mai Loi again entreated, and reminded Kabir that what the king had done was a tremendous service to them. She could not even for a moment believe that the king was not deserving of spiritual initiation. "The best way to prove it to yourself is to do what I ask you to do," Kabir replied, "and thereafter come and tell me what you hear from his mouth. Please go on to the roof of the house and, as the king walks outside, throw the entire garbage of the house upon his head."

Mai Loi did as she was asked, and threw the trash and garbage on the head of the king. "If this were my palace," he said indignantly, "no one would dare do this to me." Mai Loi returned to Kabir and repeated what the king had said.

"Didn't I tell you that the king was not yet fully deserving of the great gift of Nam?" Kabir asked.

So another six years passed by, during which the king worked as hard as he had during the first six years. And one day Kabir said to his wife, "The vessel is now ready."

"I don't find any difference in the nature of the king, whether six years ago or now," Mai Loi replied.

"If you want to see the difference," Kabir told her, "you may once again throw the garbage and rotted rubbish of the house upon the king's head."

The next day, when the king was just outside the house, she did exactly as she was asked. Upon receiving this "gift," the king looked up and said, "May you, the doer of this, live long. This mind of mine was still full of ego and self—it had to be treated this way."

Again Mai Loi related the king's words to her husband. This time Kabir replied, "As I told you, there is nothing lacking in him now."

Kabir then told the king, "Your devotion is complete now; you may go anywhere you like."

The purer the mind, the more beautiful and powerful is the soul.

What grudge does the goldsmith bear the lump of gold when he beats it with his hammer? He frees it from all blemishes, so its true beauty might shine.

—Dadu Dayal

This isn't to say we should in any way torture the body on our quest for spiritual liberation—merely that we must learn to temper the senses, tame the ego, and purify the mind. Through self-discipline, trust in our intuition, and patience with this sure but gradual process, we will have the blissful experience of Divine Love. We will know the joy of selfless service and the inner power of real humility. This practice is absolutely necessary if the soul is to be truly free.

> *We must learn to temper the senses, tame the ego, and purify the mind.*

Mind Control

Throughout the ages many have attempted to control the mind by torturing their bodies. They have slept on beds of nails. They have burned, bled, whipped, and even castrated themselves to gain supremacy over the mind. These extreme actions and ascetic practices have proved futile, for the mind cannot be tamed or controlled by them. Nor do any of these methods lead to the freedom of the soul. The masters of the Sound Current say the wild and fickle nature of the mind is subdued, however, once it has heard and experienced the bliss of the Divine Voice or Celestial Melody within. This may be experienced as a gradual unfoldment or in a moment of divine revelation, largely depending on the consciousness of the jiva (student of spirit).

An amusing story told by the Eastern mystics metaphorically illustrates the futility of some methods used to control one's mind. One day a village woman, after baking some pies, went to a nearby market to get some vegetables. She left the pies on a windowsill to cool. On the veranda of her house were her pets, a goat and a monkey, tied with ropes to the railing of the veranda. The monkey, seeing that the woman had gone out, unfastened the rope around its neck. It then ran over to the pies and helped itself to a little personal feast. Then it unfastened the rope around the goat's neck, and refastened the rope around its own.

When the woman returned home, she found that all the pies had been eaten. Going to the veranda, she saw the monkey well fastened, presenting a picture of innocence, while the goat was loose, wandering around the yard. Upset, she grabbed a stick and beat the goat. Then a neighbor, who had witnessed the whole scenario, revealed to her the actual facts of the incident.

In this allegory the monkey represents the mind, and the goat, the physical human body. The obvious inference is that the physical body is a mere instrument of the mind, and it is the mind—not the body—that is the guilty one. Keeping extreme fasts, exposing oneself to intense heat and cold, and resorting to other ascetic practices is can be likened to punishing the wrong party, while the mischievous mind remains perfectly safe as the deranged music conductor of our "body-orchestra."

So, before we can effectively create harmony within the body, we must learn to discipline and control the mind. Only then will the soul gain freedom from the negative and obsessive tendencies of the mind, and take its rightful place as the "conductor" of the mind and body.

Love, Devotion, and Surrender

Many spiritual philosophies and practices state that the destruction of the ego is necessary before making real spiritual progress. Although the ego or individuated self may stand in the way of the liberation and oneness of our soul, ego destruction is not the solution. Until a certain level of consciousness is reached, we need the ego to give us the concentrated focus and impetus to "meet spirit halfway," so to speak. The ego may be surrendered, rather than destroyed. What's the difference? How do we achieve this?

> *The ego may be surrendered, rather than destroyed.*

The answers lie in loving and accepting the ego, as it is a part of ourselves. We mustn't hate, resist, or destroy any part of ourselves; we must love and accept all facets of ourselves. This does not mean that we shouldn't change, heal, or transform certain aspects of ourselves—only that we must love them first. Love is the most healing and potent power in the universe.

This principle may be observed from a unique perspective in the following story.

There once was a gardener who diligently tended to the various plants and flowers in his garden. Every day he would see to it that his "children" got the necessary attention, water, sunlight, pruning, and so forth, necessary for their growth and health.

One day a passerby noticed the gardener tending to a small, young plant. The passing stranger remarked to his associate, "Look at that ignorant gardener—he's watering the weeds along with his little plant. At that rate, his whole garden will be overrun with weeds." They both chuckled cynically and continued walking. Meanwhile, the gardener, oblivious to the criticism of the passerby, continued his watering of the young seedling.

A few days later, the same man was walking past the garden and again noticed the gardener watering the small plant. This time he shouted to the gardener, "Don't you realize that you're watering the weeds as well as that plant? Soon the weeds will overrun everything!" The man then asked, "Why don't you simply pull out those weeds?"

The gardener calmly looked up and smiled at the stranger, saying, "This young seedling is delicate, yet gaining strength every day. It needs the weeds right now and could be damaged by rooting them out." He went on to explain, "The wild weeds pose no threat as of yet. When the plant grows stronger and larger, I'll then remove the weeds with no risk to the plant."

> *Love the weeds as well as the flowers, the mind and ego as well as the soul and spirit.*

This little tale may be seen as a metaphor for our soul's relationship with the ego. The seedling represents the soul and its development; the weeds are the ego and its manifestations. The gardener (master) knows that the soul needs the ego until it can function independently, and there is no present threat from the weeds (ego) as the gardener will safely remove them at the appropriate time. The water, sunlight, and caring of the gardener could be seen as the sound, light, and love that constantly nourish and support the soul.

Everything is purposeful and serves the "Whole." Let us love the weeds as well as the flowers, the mind and ego as well as the soul and spirit. Let us love the passersby, cynics, and critics as we love our friends and families. Let us see, feel, and love the Oneness we all share. Let us love ourselves into the fullness of the Whole. Let us truly love.

The mind and ego naturally and effortlessly surrender in the presence of this type of Love.

Tips for Staying on Your Path

Real freedom and the transcendence of the soul are only achieved with vigilant self-awareness and discipline, unflinching self-honesty, surrender to the spiritual power of love, divine grace, and devotion to the Sacred Sound within. This is the way to true mastership of body, mind, and spirit.

Self-Awareness Exercise/Questions

Before addressing the spiritual relevance of rhe Sound Current in the next chapter, I'd like to share with you a practical self-awareness exercise that has served me well over the years in helping me stay on my path. It's a great "reality check." I hope that it may serve and empower you, as well. Although I have stumbled more times than I can count, in order to keep my mind disciplined, the purpose of my soul before me, and my actions:

1. Is my choice of action motivated by love or fear?

2. Do my body, heart, and intuition resonate with this decision?

3. Does my action facilitate my moving toward my purpose and highest good, or away from them?

4. If I were to perform this action in the physical presence of the person (living or dead) that I most love, admire, and respect, how would I feel? Would the action feel appropriate?

≈

Waking From the Dream

As discussed previously, it is not possible to fully grasp spiritual concepts and truths with the finite mind. So in our present state, how do we discern the difference between reality and illusion? How do we truly know if we are dreaming? Using the conscious mind to understand the superconscious is similar to comprehending conscious reality while unconscious during sleep. While in the dream state we are convinced that it is real. Our dilemma may point to the need for a guide or teacher who has traveled those inner roads and experienced the super-consciousness of Divine Spirit.

For example, imagine yourself sleeping as a child, and your father trying to wake you up for school. You are dreaming about being a cowboy and trying to round up a herd of horses. In a semi-conscious state you say to your father, "I have to catch all the horses first." Your father lovingly but firmly says, "You have to get up now; I'll finish rounding up the horses for you." Did your father really round up the horses, or did he lie to you?

You may perceive your father as lying in this scenario, but he is speaking to you from a higher level of awareness than yours, and he has your best interests in mind. This allegory represents our experience of this so-called "conscious life."

We need to trust in someone. But only the true mystics and spiritual masters of the Sound Current know the "higher road," for they have traveled it. And they return to lovingly assist us in making the glorious journey from spiritually unconscious to superconscious and Spiritually Realized. They humbly support us in shifting our trust from the "limiting mind" to the unlimited soul-self, so that we may experience our Infinite Source.

In the next chapter, we will explore some of the secrets of the Inner Overtone and Celestial Voice within that guide us to this Source.

The Golden Horn

Once upon a time in a faraway land, a wise old king lived in a magnificent castle. His prize possession was a magical golden horn displayed in a glass case in the king's royal court.

Every day the king's guests would come from miles around to see the beautiful golden instrument. On the luckiest of days the guests would be treated to the magical and uplifting tones of the wondrous horn when the king was in the mood to play it. It was said that the sound of the golden horn could heal the body and illuminate the soul.

On one dark night, a thief sneaked past the palace guards and stole the precious horn. Eluding the guards, he escaped into the nearby mountains and hid in a cave.

After regaining his breath and composure, the thief anxiously placed the horn to his lips and began to play it. A stream of fractured and dissonant tones was released, filling the cave with a frightful sound. The harder the thief tried to improve upon the sound, the worse it sounded.

Than an extraordinary thing occurred. From deep within the cacophony he began to hear what sounded like a voice. The robber listened intently as, to his amazement, the voice of the king emerged through the reverberations.

"I visit you in order to bestow my blessings and gratitude upon you," said the king.

The thief stood frozen, in awe and disbelief.

"You have greatly helped me to release my attachment to the outer manifestations of sound and matter. For this I thank you.

"I believed that I was free when I discovered the golden horn, but learned I was not. Then I thought I was free when I played its tones, but found I was only more deeply attached to its mystery.

"Every day of my life I played the horn. While learning to master its mellifluous tones, I also learned to hear its healing and transcendent message. At last this day has come, when its music became so beautiful that you stole it. In passing it on to you, with an open heart, I am released. I am now blessed with the bliss of hearing the Divine Melody within.

"You now possess the Golden Horn of Truth. When you play it, whatever is in your heart will be revealed. You cannot express its beauty by playing it with calculation, pride and ego. You cannot access its healing power by trying to control it, or by pretending that you have it.

"The power of the Golden Horn is expressed and made manifest only through the purity of the vibrations in the one who plays it. And its magic is revealed by the awareness of those who receive it. Devote yourself to that which gives it resonance."

(((((22)))))

The Inner Overtone or Sacred Sound Current

*In the beginning was the Word, and the Word
was with God, and the Word was God.*

—St. John

This Word is not, as is usually believed, a written word. Actually, it is a power that emanates continuously from the Supreme Being, the Power that created and now sustains the vast universe of universes.

The saints and perfect masters teach their disciples how to contact this power, which is everywhere present…and is heard by initiates as the most enchanting and enrapturing harmony or melody. This music is not only beautiful, it is also purifying and uplifting. It purifies the human mind, and then draws the soul upwards with an irresistible Power—the Power of Love of the Supreme God Himself.

—Maharaj Sawan Singh

For ages mystics and sages have made reference to the Sacred Sound or Celestial Melody that can be found within every one of us. It is the eternal, primordial Sound, which, emanating from Divine Loving Consciousness or God, manifests and sustains creation. It is a holistic Sound reverberating throughout the entirety of existence and resonating in every cell of the human body, giving us life and consciousness.

The real Masters of the Sound Current are those who have achieved the ultimate and highest spiritual state of consciousness through meditation on this Divine Sound within while still resident in the physical body. On the spiritual plane, these masters are One. They have traversed the many inner regions of sound, light, love, and spirit—humbly and lovingly offering us the benefit of their wisdom and direct experience. When a spiritual seeker is ready, the master reveals the secrets of the Inner Overtone or Sound Current and the means by which we may return "home" on it.

When I was only 22 years old, I received this great blessing from the late Sound Current Master Huzur Charan Singh Ji, who made his transition in 1990. This profound experience—and my subsequent study and meditation—dramatically changed my life. The ancient teachings of the masters, along with the principles of sound and vibration, made perfect sense at the time and inspired me to direct my life's path and personal frequency toward prioritizing my inner spiritual life. These efforts also greatly changed my perspective on my outer life. The results were that most of the "burning questions" I'd always had about life were answered. I developed a deeper relationship with myself and God. And I learned (not always easily) about the beauty of simplicity and profound healing power of love. Many other lessons learned in my meditations and healings are mentioned throughout this book.

Sound Symbols and Instruments

The outer instruments of sound can be seen as imitations of and a metaphor for the pure, inner sounds. For example, the ringing of bells is mentioned in the scriptures of all religions. Bells hang from domes within Buddhist and Hindu temples. Whoever enters the temple rings a bell. In the human head, which is also similar to a dome, one may hear the Inner Overtone or Divine Melody. In the same manner, Christian churches have high steeples in which a bell is hung. These are based on the shape of the nose. In the human body, "temple of the living God," when the soul is concentrated at a point between the two eyebrows, the "seat of the soul," one hears the sound of the bell.

In *Healing with Sound and Music*, Hazrat Inayat Khan writes, "The secret of the continual ringing of the bell practiced by the churches of all times, even now, is that it is not only a bell to call people, it is to tune them up to their tone. It was to suggest, 'There is a tone going on in you, get yourself tuned to it!'"

> *This enchanting bell sound is one of many sonorous manifestations of the Sound Current.*

This enchanting bell sound is one of many sonorous manifestations of the Sound Current. As the soul-consciousness evolves, develops, and rises up through the "many mansions" of spiritual awareness, the inner sounds seem to change and evolve as well. Although hundreds of different sounds may be heard—thunder, whistle, violin, drum—in actuality, there is but One Divine Sound that emanates a bell-like sound. This is first experienced indirectly as an echo of an echo of an echo. This is in accordance with the level of the soul's spiritual development. Eventually, by holding the focus of attention at the seat of the soul, or "eye center" within the forehead, the soul is vibrationally cleansed of its impurities and is able to hear the True Sound in all its infinite resonance.

Masters of the Sound Current

Rituals and rites...the ceremonial parts of every religion differ according to the customs of the age, and climates and conditions of the countries; but the real Essence of Truth, the Spirituality at the foundation of all religions is the same. They all lead us to the Holy Sound, the Word, the Logos, by hearing which we attain salvation.

—Maharaj Charan Singh

Light on Sant Mat

The true "mystic mentors" and Masters of the Sound Current selflessly offer their support in helping us understand and utilize this Divine Vibration to elevate our consciousness and liberate our souls. But do we listen to them? Do we appreciate the value of their wisdom and experience, or are we too caught up in our own worlds to recognize the wonderful gifts they bring us?

It may be difficult for us to be fully receptive to these gifts because of our many influences, such as family upbringing, religious background, and cultural and socio-political pressures. In addition to these and other issues, there is our own personal nature, psychological makeup, intellect, emotional needs, and so on.

And with the limited time available to most of us, it becomes quite difficult to always make informed choices—choices that may even dramatically change our lives. But who has the time to study every spiritual and philosophical view, every bit of scientific research, all facts of history—or even all the income tax laws?

This is why we consult with experts in particular fields of interest. If we wish to become adept at business, medicine, law, or sports, would we not study with experts in those fields who have experienced and mastered the methodologies, shortcuts, and techniques for achieving success in those particular areas?

It is no different in the realms of sound, light, love, and spirit. The Masters of the Sound Current have experienced and mastered these important inner aspects of soul consciousness and are always available to us, as they say, "When the student is ready...." These mystic mentors have made the inner journey through dimensions of "ringing radiance" and pure spiritual Reality, and have returned to avail themselves to us— to show us how to do the same.

However, when it comes to matters such as spirituality, one's deepest fears sometimes emerge. Whether these fears are embedded in our consciousness by our parents, by religious leaders, or by society in general, we need to overcome them if we are to be truly free. And although study and knowledge are obviously useful tools, experience serves us even better. Our sometimes obsessive need to control and know too much contributes to our dilemma, as well. One of my favorite stories told by the mystics aptly illustrates this predicament.

> *The Masters of the Sound Current have experienced and mastered these important inner aspects of soul consciousness.*

A blind man was walking along and fell into a deep well. Another man happened to pass that way and, taking pity on the sad condition of the blind man, offered to help free him. For this purpose, he dropped one end of a long rope into the well and asked the blind man to catch hold of it, so that he could be pulled out.

Instead of taking hold of the rope, however, the blind man started a long and senseless rant, asking, "How could I have fallen into such a deep well, and what guarantee do I have that I will not fall into some other well as soon as I get out?"

The patient and caring helper replied, "It would be in your best interest, to take hold of the rope so that you may be freed. You can always study the details of the situation later."

The man in the well then suspiciously asked, "Why do you want to take me out of here, and what motive do you have for helping me?"

By now, the patience of the kind rescuer was wearing thin by all this nonsense, but he calmly replied, "You need to grab hold of the rope now if you wish to be pulled from this well."

Again, however, the blind man continued to ramble on, "How is it that you did not fall into the well?" The rescuer, now at the end of his rope, told him he had other important tasks to attend to, so he would have to leave the blind man in the well if he did not come out within a few minutes.

"All right," said the blind man. "But first please tell me, how deep is this well, and when was it built?"

"Well, it's deep enough to be the grave of many like you," said the rescuer, and he went on his way.

Isn't this what we all do, in one way or another? Are we open and receptive to the opportunities available that can truly liberate us, or do we overanalyze the situation? Can we become so self-involved and fearful that we may lose all objectivity and trust in others? Is our intellect and reasoning put to the best use, or do they sometimes become great obstacles that impede our true freedom and transformation? How can we know the **Truth?**

The answers to these and all other questions lie within us. We need only go inside and find them.

Spiritual Sound

The Masters of the Sound Current tell us "spiritual sound" is not an easy subject matter for speech or writing; it needs to be experienced to be fully understood. However, the Great Master (as he was lovingly referred to by thousands of his devotees in India and elsewhere) Maharaj Sawan Singh (1858–1948) profoundly wrote in his book series, *Philosophy of the Masters*:

> The soul-current of consciousness originates from the Lord and pervades everything. It gives life to the whole of the creation and can take every living being back to his (or her) Original Home. The Lord creates and sustains the entire universe through this great Current of Power. The currents of the Lord pervade everywhere, like radio waves. His divine music fills all space. Unless we are correctly tuned to it we cannot hear this music. As we grow more and more subtle, we begin to hear clearly its melodies. Shabd (Spiritual Sound) is a string that connects everyone and everything with the Lord.... Like electricity, Shabd, whether manifest or unmanifest, pervades everywhere. It is all-powerful and is the Creator of all.

When translated accurately, the scriptures of all religions reveal Spiritual Sound as the Creator of the universe. The spiritual masters of India refer to it as Shabda or Shabd (word, inner sound, or song), Dhun (manifestation of Shabd), Nam (name, Shabd, or Word), Anahad or Anahat Shabd (unstruck or limitless sound), or Nad (inner melody or music) of the Vedas; Nada (the soundless sound) of the Upanishads; the Word, Name, Logos, Holy Ghost, Holy Spirit, or Living Water of the Bible; the Bang-i-asmani (sound of the skies), the Kalam or Kalma (word or sound), Kalam-i-ilahi (word of God) in the Koran; the Sarosh (sound) of the Zoroastrians; the Akashvani (voice or music of the sky) or Dev Vani (celestial voice) of the Hindu scriptures; and the Divya Dhwani (divine sound) of the Jains.

> *"Spiritual sound"*
> *is not an easy*
> *subject matter for*
> *speech or writing; it*
> *needs to be*
> *experienced to be*
> *fully understood.*

Madame Blavatsky, founder of the Theosophical Society, described the Divine Sound as the "Voice of the Silence." In the Masonic Order this Logos is described as the "Lost Word," which is sought after by every Masonic Master. Buddhism knows it as Fohat, or the "sonorous light of the Logos." In Tibetan Buddhism it is related to the Bardol Thodol, and Chinese mysticism refers to it as Kwan-Yin-Tien or the Melodious Heaven of Sound. Lao Tzu described the Tao, meaning the Way or the Word, as "unimpeded harmony," and the source of all things. He also wrote about the Great Tone "that goes beyond all usual imagination." The Persian Sufis called it Wadan, the Divine Sound. The Sufi Saint, Hazrat Inayat Khan, who had access to the spiritual regions, describes the Sound as Divine Music. He said everything manifested from It and Its manifestation.

More Words on the Word

Archaeological excavations in Egypt have shown that King Ikhnaton, who ruled about 4,000 years ago, encouraged inner sound practice (then called Aton). In Egyptian cosmogony it is Thoth, the Divine Intelligence, who uttered Words that form the world. The ancient Greek philosophers also mentioned the Sound Current. Socrates stated that he heard within him sound that took him to indescribable spiritual regions. Plato also mentioned it. Pythagoras called it the "music of the spheres." It is called Logos (the Word) in Greek. It is also synonymous with Patanjali's OM. Other terms used include Hu, Udgit, Audible Life Stream, Ringing Radiance,

Infinite Frequency, Limitless Vibration, Celestial Melody, Inner Music, Song or Tone, Divine Voice or Word, and Eternal, Holy or Sacred Sound.

Persian saint Shams-i-Tabriz, from the 12th and 13th centuries, said: "From the Sound (Word) the entire creation came into being, all light emanated from it."

In Sikhism's holy book, the *Granth Sahib*, possibly the most complete scripture available today, the terms *Unstruck Melody* and *Word* are often used to refer to the Sound Current: "Blessed, blessed am I, that my God is my Spouse. Within whose court ringeth the Unstruck Melody (of the Word). Night and day, I abide in joy, hearing ever the Music of Bliss: Yea, no more in this state is pain or sorrow, neither birth nor death."

Great yet humble 15th-century poet Saint Kabir wrote extensively of spiritual devotion and the mysterious "Unstruck Music," which delivers the soul into an enraptured state:

> There falls the rhythmic beat of life and death: Rapture wells forth, and all space is radiant with light. There the Unstruck Music is sounded; it is the music of the three worlds.
>
> There millions of lamps of sun and moon are burning: There the drum beats, and the lover swings in play. There love-songs resound, and light rains in showers; and the worshiper is entranced in the taste of the heavenly nectar.

Elsewhere in one of his poems Kabir writes: "Says Kabir, realize the Shabd, O brother, for Shabd is the Creator himself."

Likewise, in the 20th century, Sawan Singh wrote of this Sacred Sound:

> The Shabd is conscious and consciousness. It is a wave of the ocean of the Lord and a man is a particle of His Being. He is related to Him as a part is related to the whole. The Lord is the ocean of super-consciousness, and Shabd is its wave. The soul is a drop of this ocean. The wave of super-consciousness or Shabd attracts the conscious soul toward it and absorbs it. Until the soul, with the help of the Shabd, rises to its Original Home, it cannot achieve salvation. The melody of the Shabd is ringing within us. When the soul is connected with it, it becomes fit to rise from the finite toward the infinite.

Etheric Vibrations

In *The Path of The Masters*, Dr. Julian Johnson refers to the Shabd as the Audible Life Stream, and describes it as "the essence and life of all things." He writes:

> When any man speaks in this world, he simply sets in motion atmospheric vibrations. But when God speaks, he not only sets in motion etheric vibrations but he himself moves in and through those vibrations. In truth it is God himself that vibrates all through infinite space. God is not static, latent: He is superlatively dynamic. When he speaks, everything in existence vibrates, and that is the Sound, the Shabd; and it can be heard by the inner ear, which has been trained to hear it. It is the Divine energy in process of manifestation that is the holy Shabd. It is in fact the only way in which the Supreme One can be seen and heard—this mighty, luminous and musical wave creating and enchanting.

Scientists have affirmed that, from a vibrational perspective, all that is in the Universe is present in man. In fact, man is a vibrational reality of sound, light, and form, the different states of which are only differences in frequencies or vibrations. The Universe is the macrocosm; the body the microcosm.

Divine Sound in the Bible

There are numerous references to the Divine Sound in the Bible. For example, the book of Revelation (14:2) says: "And I heard a voice from Heaven like the sound of many waters and like the sound of loud thunder; the voice I heard was like the sound of harpers playing on their harps."

Man is a vibrational reality of sound, light, and form.

Late philologist and archaeologist Edmund Bordeaux Szekely, cofounder of the International Biogenic Society, came upon secret Aramaic texts in the Vatican, which date back to the third century after the death of Jesus. Szekely translated a revealing document called the "Essene Gospel of Peace" in which the following appears: "In the beginning was the Sound, and the Sound was with God, and the Sound was God."

After almost 20 years of meticulous research, Dr. Szekely became convinced that Jesus was a member of the highly respected Essene spiritual community and therefore would have had intimate knowledge of their spiritual tradition. As he relates in *The Essene Jesus*, "There was the Essene Brotherhood at the Dead Sea which planted The Essene Tree of Life, whose highest branch was represented by the Essene Jesus."

Concentration on the Primordial Sound

Madame Blavatsky, author of *The Secret Doctrine* and *The Voice of Silence*, writes of "the primordial Sound that flows outward and downward to create and sustain the entire system of universes, of which man is the microcosm." She also said, "Students in the West have little or no idea of the forces that lie in Sound." The opening verses of *The Voice of Silence* state, "He who would hear the voice of Nada, 'the Soundless Sound,' and comprehend it, he has to learn the nature of Dharana (concentration)."

The art of concentration is an exact, all-encompassing discipline that is necessary for the practice of "sound current yoga" or meditation, the means by which we connect with Divine Sound. On the supreme current of the Word or Shabd we descended into the human form, and by that same current we shall ascend to our primal Source. Ultimately, it is up to us to choose when and where we wish to focus our attention and energy. Are we ready to reawaken in ourselves a new spiritual perception and journey on the inner path of the Sound Current and Divine Word?

> *Our attention does not catch the Sound Current because the attention is saturated with the world of matter.*

Because this Infinite Overtone emanates from within the body, this is where we need to concentrate our attention. Toning with the voice begins the concentration process and deepens our conscious connection with sound. During meditation the repetition of mantras or sacred words that correspond to inner, spiritual planes occupies and focuses the mind in preparation for ascension. Then, by opening the heart of the soul with loving intention and spiritual longing, the magnificence of the Celestial Melody is finally realized. For the first time, we experience the infinite nature of sound, light, and love, and become a vehicle for the healing, uplifting power of Sacred Sound.

Inverting the Attention

I die daily.

—St. Paul

Taming the "wild" mind and reversing the downward flow of its attention is, admittedly, no easy task. But it is necessary if we wish to reap the wondrous rewards of Spirit that lie within us. We must, temporarily, shut off or "die" to the outer world so that we may become aware of or reborn to the inner world.

The masters tell us that the soul is covered by mind and matter. Our attention does not catch the Sound Current because the attention is saturated with matter or the world of matter. After reaching the eye center, we will have washed away all matter and then be fit to catch the Current. Reaching the eye center is a prerequisite to catching the Current. The eye center could be seen as an inter-dimensional doorway or portal through which the soul passes in deep states of meditation and at the time of death.

Withdrawing and inverting our attention is a gradual process requiring patience and determination. The masters use the analogy that our attention is sticking to the body and material world as if it were a fine silk cloth entangled in a prickly, thorny shrub. If one were to pull the cloth forcibly, the cloth would be torn to pieces. But if one patiently and gently disentangles it from each thorn, one at a time, one can succeed in removing the cloth intact.

Similarly, we need to use patience and gentleness, combined with concentration, in practicing the withdrawal of our attention. However, it is common to encounter some inner resistance while attempting to tackle the mind with the "attention-inversion" process.

An amusing story I heard many years ago may shed some light on the situation. There was an old lady standing under a street light outside her house one evening. She was looking down at the ground as if looking for something. A passerby noticed her and also began looking down for whatever she may have dropped. He asked the woman what she had lost, and she replied that it was her keys. They both continued their search but could see no keys anywhere. After a few more minutes the man asked the old lady if she had any idea where the keys might be located. "Oh yes," she replied. "I'm sure they are in my house."

Stopped in his tracks, the perplexed man asked, "If your keys are in your house, then why are you looking for them out here?"

To this she replied, "It's too dark in there!"

This little tale may help illustrate our hesitancy to practice meditation and turn our attention within. Perhaps we are not convinced that there is light within the darkness. Maybe the process of "going within" taps into a primal fear of the dark. Perhaps we are simply too impatient. However, any resistance we may be holding must be overcome if we are to pierce the veil and enter the inner regions of light and sound.

Light and Sound

If thine eye be single thy whole body shall be full of light.

—Luke (17:21)

A light is shining within each one of us behind the eyes, and a sweet melodious music emanates from its light.

—Spiritual Discourses

The Masters of the Sound Current teach us that there are two mediums by which we can perceive and experience the Inner Overtone and Sacred Tone; they are light and sound, the essence of our soul-self. It is through light and sound that we are heaven-bound.

> *It is through light and sound that we are heaven-bound.*

Independent of our physical senses, the soul itself has a seeing and hearing capacity. The mystics call the soul's seeing faculty **nirat**, and its hearing faculty **surat**. Through the nirat, the soul can perceive the brilliant radiance of tremendous Light within. Through the surat, the soul can perceive the profound power of the Celestial Sound. This perceptive process aligns one with the practice of the purest and highest form of yoga (spiritual exercises leading to the union of the soul with God), referred to as Surat Shabd Yoga (the spiritual practice by which the consciousness is applied to the hearing of the Divine Word or Sound Current within).

In *Philosophy of the Masters,* Maharaj Sawan Singh describes the soul's ascension and liberation with sound and light:

> All the great souls, whether of the East or the West, who went inside and had access to the inner regions, have mentioned the Sound and the Light. The soul is imprisoned in the cage of the mind and the body. Both light and sound

are within us. The Sound and Light are related to the two faculties of the soul namely Surat (hearing) and Nirat (seeing). Surat hears and Nirat sees. In ascending upward through the spiritual regions, Nirat leads and Surat follows. After the maturing of the Surat (the soul's power of hearing) and of Nirat (the soul's power of seeing) the soul is freed from the bondage of the body and rises to the higher regions.

Regarding differences in various forms of yoga, Sound Current Master Maharaj Charan Singh says, in *Light on Sant Mat*:

> Hatha Yoga, I may point out, is an excellent discipline for the body. Raja Yoga is better but that too does not enable you to control the mind fully nor does it finish your series of births and deaths, for the seeds of karma are not destroyed by that method. Surat Shabd Yoga enables you to "roast" the seeds of karmas, as it were, so that they cannot sprout again. Mind can only be fully controlled by a Power which has its origin beyond the mind, and that is the Divine Sound.

In his book *Spiritual Gems*, Sawan Singh states, "The highest and easiest method that the greatest sages of different countries have followed and preached, for the liberation of the soul, is the path of Surat Shabd Yoga—which for want of a better word in the English language is usually translated as 'Sound Current.'"

And, from *Philosophy of the Masters*:

> Surat Shabd Yoga is very ancient and has existed from the very beginning. It is natural. One cannot add to or subtract anything from it. The Shabd was in the beginning. It created this universe. The soul has a natural affinity for the Heavenly Music of Nam....The benefits of practicing Surat Shabd Yoga are very great. The inner melody and light appear and one comes to know the True Reality.

The Eye Center

The masters teach that the access point to the Sound Current, in the body, is at the "eye center" or "eye focus." This point is located between the eyebrows, just above and behind the physical eyes. It is also called the

"10th door" or " 10th gate," because it is one of the 10 apertures or portals within the body.

A significant difference between this portal and the other nine, however, is that the other portals (seven in the head and two below) are physical and sense-based, and the 10th is non-physical and etheric. The lower nine apertures carry the flow of attention and vibrational energy downward and outward into the world and its related objects. With the concentration of attention at the eye center or 10th door, the vibrational flow is directed inward and upward, allowing the soul-consciousness to connect with the Inner Overtone. This process represents the purest and highest form of meditation and, as the masters say, allows the soul to ultimately return to its True Home.

Closing the nine doors, one finds liberation
at the tenth, there ever resonates the
limitless melody of the Word.

—Guru Nanak, *The Adi Granth*

The masters say the soul's journey within the Sound Current really begins at the eye center and proceeds upward from there. They say, "If you want to get to the roof of a building and you are on the second floor, why go down to the basement first?" In other words, why waste time in the body's lower chakras if you want to return to your true, spiritual Home? Though there may be some benefits gained by focusing on various chakras for healing, and though concentration is strengthening and developing, they say the real spiritual practice starts at the eye center.

The real spiritual practice starts at the eye center.

It is not so much a technique that stimulates the nirat and surat, as it is the uplifting spiritual power intrinsically contained within the soul's longing, love, and devotion for its Source. But the spiritual practice itself requires trust, patience, faith, and, above all, one-pointed attention. How many of us can easily withdraw our attention from the worldly pursuits and pleasures, and patiently redirect it within on a daily basis? Now, that's a spiritual reality check, but it is also what the masters say is required if we are serious about developing super-consciousness and "building our treasure in heaven."

In this context, another inspiring message from the great Master of the Sound Current, Maharaj Sawan Singh:

> The supreme Lord, the soul and the Shabd are a holy Trinity. The One Lord exists in all the three forms. The soul has no separate existence from the timeless Being. It is a particle of Him.
>
> By practicing the Shabd all diseases, vices and sins are removed.... [O]ne becomes very pure and completely detached. Shabd is the support of life and death. The fear of death is banished.... [O]ne crosses the ocean of worldly existence.
>
> By the practice of the Sound, light appears within and the Lotus of the heart blossoms. One realizes his true Self and attains the state of dying while living. He transcends the domain of...time. He goes into trance in the Void, and the tenth door opens. He learns the sign of the Lord's door. He is dyed in the hue of the Lord, and true devotion and Divine bliss arise within him. He is honored in the Court of the Lord. He attains salvation and realizes the most blissful state.

Total Freedom

The true spiritual saints and masters do not come to teach us how to improve the world, but to help us to free ourselves from it. This is not escapism, but practical applied spirituality. They teach us how to transcend our temporal finite existence and prepare for the infinite experience. It is not pessimism to recognize and accept that there has never ever been peace and harmony in the world, nor will there ever be. This is not the purpose of this transitory and illusionary dimension, according to the masters. If there ever really was peace on earth, we wouldn't want to leave here and return home to our Divine Heritage. The masters say this is a "training ground" to prepare us for the Real life—eternal life of pure love and bliss. This is true optimism and Realism.

My "mystic mentor," Huzur Maharaj Charan Singh, used to tell the following story.

In a prison there is a large number of prisoners. A kindhearted philanthropist goes to the prison and pays for the supply of fresh, cold water for the inmates every day during the hot summer. He has certainly done a very good thing for the prisoners, because he has given them something refreshing to drink instead of the stale, warm water they were previously receiving.

Another noble and kindhearted philanthropist then goes to the prison and, finding that the inmates are getting very poor food, provides them with delicious meals, which they enjoy very much. He has also done a very good thing for the prisoners.

Then a third kindhearted philanthropist goes to the prison and, seeing that during the freezing cold winter the inmates have no warm clothing, spends a large sum of money that provides them with woolen clothes. He has also done a great good deed, possibly exceeding that of the other two charitable men.

Taking pity on the inmates, all three benefactors have done their best to improve the inmates' living conditions. From C-class prisoners, they have become A-class prisoners, and their life in prison has been made much more comfortable and far less insufferable. But in spite of help from the philanthropists, the inmates were still prisoners and had to remain in the jail.

Then a fourth kindhearted man goes to the prison. He has the key to the prison, and he opens its gates and sets the prisoners free forever. Thus, the kindness and generosity of the fourth man was of the greatest value.

Similarly, the Masters of Sound hold the key to this vast prison we live in, offering us total freedom. They help release us for all time by freely sharing the vibrational secrets for returning to our real Home. As long as the soul does not go back and merge with its Source, we can never escape from the prison of the body or the suffering and misery of this world. Therefore, the value of the help given by the Masters of the Sound Current is far greater than that of any charitable person, social reformer, or political leader.

Spiritual Activism

Our reality, as we experience it, may be seen as similar to the experience of watching a movie in a theater. Before entering the theater we make an agreement with ourselves to suspend disbelief for a couple of hours, or the length of the film. As we watch the movie, any number of emotions may be felt—some joyful and uplifting; others perhaps painful and depressing. We may be captivated on various levels of involvement. But if we feel aghast and offended by something that is occurring on the screen, it is not likely that we would suddenly try to tear the screen down or chop it up with a machete. (It wouldn't stop the projection anyway.) This is because we know that what's going on in the movie is not real and that our suspension of disbelief is for the purpose of enjoying the film experience.

When it comes to enjoying and living in this world, however, we have forgotten that it is not real, and that we once made a similar agreement to temporarily experience this dimension of pleasure and pain. We have forgotten our real Home of infinite love, joy, and bliss.

In the movie theater, if we want to put an end to the horrific images being projected on the screen, all we need do is go into the projection room and extract the film or projector. The projection then ceases; the movie is over. Similarly, if and when we tire of the terrible pain, suffering, intolerance, and injustices of the world—in the "big picture"—it does little good trying to change the external effects of projections from the collective consciousness.

> *More effective is being an "inner activist" and a "spiritual warrior" of the Sound Current.*

Outer activism is akin to destroying a film screen: The effects are minimal and temporary. More effective is being an "inner activist" and a "spiritual warrior" of the Sound Current. Prove this to yourself by accessing the "main projection room" located right inside your own forehead at the eye center. This active participation will give you access to the creative consciousness. But most importantly, this form of activism will give you the means for changing your reality with the Divine Infinite Overtone. This "spiritual activism" creates the most effective and permanent results.

Going Home

The greatest lesson of the Overtone is to
resonate with all, to know all, and be silent.

—Wayne Perry

For aspiring mystics and inner-sound-searchers wishing to access the Sound Current, the best preparation is to follow the various toning, listening, and meditation guidelines elaborated upon throughout this book. These self-empowering techniques will greatly assist in stilling the mind, uplifting the soul, and tuning your frequency for the reception of the Inner Overtone.

However, from ancient times to the present, real mystics have traditionally advised studying under the tutelage of a "realized" Sound Current Master. Through these experienced living examples of love and devotion we may receive the inner transmission of Sacred Sound necessary to free us from the shackles of worldly desires and attachments.

Upon hearing the Celestial Overtone and tasting the Divine Nectar within, the fleeting and temporal pleasures of the outer world lose their addictive appeal. We will then be ready for the true liberation of the soul. As they say in the East, "When the chela (student) is ready, the guru (teacher) appears."

> Tone your own pure frequency
>
> Colors you can hear, sounds that you can see
>
> Lift your voice, own your tone
>
> Feel your spirit soar when you overtone.
>
> Voices dance, notes collide
>
> Overtones expand—brilliant light inside
>
> Tone in trust, trust in Tone
>
> Time to catch the Sound—
>
> Ride the Current Home!
>
> —Wayne Perry

$$(((((\, \bullet \,)))))$$

Aftertone

I don't know if it is our role as citizens of planet Earth to try and change the world. I do believe, however, that by having the intention, commitment, wisdom, and spiritual maturity to transform ourselves by going to the "projection room" within us, we will automatically and profoundly improve the world. If enough of us access the source of the projection inside the collective consciousness, the external manifestation can't help but change. More importantly, by taking this kind of personal responsibility we will discover our true purpose by loving ourselves into our fullness.

This is the purest form of love, because, by loving our real Soul-Self, we love our Divine Source. And this pure, spiritual love enables us to see and love all others as ourselves until we fully experience the reality of our infinite Oneness. As spiritual activists, we perform the highest service— to the One. This is Real Activism.

You are not one of many; you are really many of One. I acknowledge, encourage, love, and support you, and all of my "fellow facets" and "kindred-spirit-aspects," who have the vision and courage to live compassionately in the world, yet not be of it.

Honoring yourself and others by "putting your loving where your mouth is," and your attention where your spirit is, will free you to "own your tone" and tune your soul.

Voicing Your Soul

Explore your inner depth, and you'll scale your greatest height.

Knowing-nothing-wisdom frees the needing to be right.

You can't stand for truth while clinging to the wall.

And resisting the pain won't soften your fall.

When you let yourself sit, you'll know where you stand.

Sound Medicine

You'll rise to the equation, and know how to land.
Resonate with dissonance—be silent and still,
while the world shouts and screams
why they can't have their fill.
Take charge of your thoughts—make each one your child.
Balance discipline with love and they'll never run wild.
Then, stand up for love—'cause you can't really fall,
When down is pointing upward, and the echoes leave the hall.
We haven't much time here, so make each day your best.
When you're serving the Timeless, less is more and more is less.
Your past—just a daydream, an appealing yesterday.
When no longer useful, the surface peels away.
Now, this moment's forever, if you recognize your role.
And remember your future by voicing your soul.
You can't memorize the Word, but It remembers you.
When you're the One and Only One, there's nothing left to
do...

—Wayne Perry

Bibliography

Andrews, Ted. *Sacred Sounds: Transformation through Music & Word*. St. Paul, Minn.: Llewellyn, 1996.

Bach, Richard. *Illusions.* New York: Dell Publishing, 1977.

Beaulieu, John. *Music and Sound in the Healing Arts*. Barrytown, N.Y.: Station Hill Press, 1987.

Berendt, Joachim-Ernst. *The World Is Sound: Nada Brahma.* Rochester, Vt.: Destiny Books, 1987.

Blavatsky, H.P. *The Voice of Silence*. Wheaton, Ill.: Theosophical University Press, 1889.

Campbell, Don, ed. *Music: Physician for Times to Come*. Wheaton, Ill.: Quest Books, 1991.

——. *The Roar of Silence*. Wheaton, Ill.: The Theosophical Publishing House, 1989.

Capra, Fritjof. *The Tao of Physics*. Boston: Shambhala Publications, 1999.

Chopra, Deepak, M.D. *Quantum Healing*. New York: Bantam, 1989.

——. *Perfect Health*. New York: Harmony Books, 1991.

——. *Ageless Body, Timeless Mind*. New York: Harmony Books, 1993.

Cook, John. *The Book of Positive Quotations (Compilation)*. Minneapolis, Minn.: Fairview Press, 1993.

Dewhurst-Maddock, Olivea. *The Book of Sound Therapy*. London: Fireside, 1993.

Dossey, Larry, M.D. *Healing Words*. New York: HarperCollins, 1993.

Edwards, Sharry. *Signature Sound Technologies Published Papers*. Athens, Ohio: Signature Sound Works, 1992.

Gardner-Gordon, Joy. *The Healing Voice*. Freedom, Calif.: The Crossing Press, 1993.

Garfield, Laeh Maggie. *Sound Medicine*. Berkeley, Calif.: Celestial Arts, 1987.

Gaynor, Mitchell L., M.D. *Sounds of Healing*. New York: Broadway Books, 1999.

Gundersen, P. Erik. *The Handy Physics Answer Book*. Canton, Mich.: Visible Ink Press, 1999.

Goldman, Jonathan. *Healing Sounds*. Rockport, Mass.: Element Books, 1992.

———. *Shifting Frequencies*. Flagstaff, Ariz.: Light Technology, 1998.

Hagemann, Anneliese Gabriel. *Dowsing/Divining*. Wautoma, Wis.: 3 H Dowsing International, 1998.

Jampolsky, Gerald G. *Love Is Letting Go of Fear*. New York: Bantam, 1970.

Jenny, Hans. *Cymatics: Vols. I & II*. (Video.) Basel, Switzerland: Basilius Presse, 1967, 1974.

Johari, Harish. *Chakras: Energy Centers of Transformation*. Rochester, Vt.: Destiny Books, 1987.

John-Roger, and Peter McWilliams. *You Can't Afford the Luxury of a Negative Thought*. Los Angeles: Prelude, 1988.

Johnson, Julian P. *The Path of the Masters*. Punjab, India: Radha Soami Satsang Beas, 1939.

Keyes, Laurel Elizabeth. *Toning: The Creative Power of the Voice*. Marina del Rey, Calif.: DeVorss, 1973.

Khan, Hazrat Inayat. *Healing with Sound and Music*. New Lebanon, N.Y.: Omega Publications, 1988.

———. *The Mysticism of Sound; Music: The Power of the Word; Cosmic Language (a compendium)*. London: Barrie and Rockliff, 1960.

Laskow, Leonard, M.D. *Healing with Love*. New York: HarperCollins, 1992.

Leet, Leonora. *Secret Doctrine of the Kabbalah*. Rochester, Vt.: Inner Traditions, 1999.

Leighton, Ralph. *Deep In the Heart of Tuva*. Roslyn, N.Y. : Ellipsis Arts, 1996.

Maman, Fabian. *The Role of Music in the Twenty-first Century*. Redondo Beach, Calif.: Tama-Do, 1997.

Manners, Peter Guy. *Cymatic Therapy*. Worcestershire, England: Bretforton, 1976.

Marciniak, Barbara. *Bringers of the Dawn*. Santa Fe, N.M.: Bear & Company, 1992.

Newman, Frederick R. *Mouthsounds*. New York: Workman, 1980.

Patent, Arnold M. *You Can Have It All*. Hillsboro, Oreg.: Beyond Words Publishing, 1995.

Perry, Wayne. "Musical Spheres: Sound, Color and Planetary Vibrations." *Perceptions Magazine*, Spring 1994: 51

———. *The Secrets to Healing with Sound & Toning (Recorded Media)*. West Hollywood, Calif.: Musikarma, 2002.

Pert, Candace B., Ph.D. *Molecules of Emotion*. New York.: Scribner, 1997.

Powell, John, S.J. *Unconditional Love*. Valencia, Calif.: Tabor Publishing, 1978.

Puri, Ishwar C. *Anatomy of Consciousness*. Punjab, India: Ishwar Chandra Puri, 1986.

Rael, Joseph. *Being and Vibration*. Tulsa, Okla.: Council Oak, 1993.

Sethi, V.K. *Kabir: The Weaver of God's Name*. Punjab, India: Radha Soami Satsang Beas, 1984.

Sheldrake, Rupert. *Of Sound, Mind & Body*. (VHS compilation.) Epping, N.H.: Lumina Productions, 1992.

Singh, Maharaj Charan. *Light On Sant Mat*. Punjab, India: Radha Soami Satsang Beas, 1958.

———. *Spiritual Discourses*. Punjab, India: Radha Soami Satsang Beas, 1964.

Singh, Maharaj Sawan. *Philosophy of the Masters*. Punjab, India: Radha Soami Satsang Beas, 1964.

———. *Spiritual Gems*. Punjab, India: Radha Soami Satsang Beas, 1965.

———. *Tales of the Mystic East (a compilation)*. Punjab, India: Radha Soami Satsang Beas, 1961.

Steiner, Rudolf. *The Inner Nature of Music and the Experience of Tone*. Herndon, Va.: Anthroposophic Press, 1983.

Szekely, Edmund Bordeaux. *The Essene Gospel of Peace*. Nelson, British Columbia: International Biogenic Society, 1937.

———. *The Essene Jesus*. Nelson, British Columbia: International Biogenic Society, 1978.

Thompson, Jeffrey D. Website articles on Brainwave Entrainment/ Biotuning/Sound Healing. Encintas, CA. Center for Neuroacoustic Research, 1996. *www.neuroacoustic.com*.

Tiller, William. *Radionics, Radiesthesia and Physics*. Los Altos, Calif.: Academy of Parapsychology & Medicine, 1971.

Tomatis, Alfred A. *The Conscious Ear*. Barrytown, N.Y.: Station Hill Press, 1991.

"Wayne Perry's Heart Touch Show" (FM Radio Broadcast). Los Angeles. 1992, 1993 (Sharry Edwards); 1993 (Jonathan Goldman); 1994 (Jeffrey D. Thompson).

White, J. Stanley. *Liberation of the Soul*. Punjab, India: Radha Soami Satsang Beas, 1972.

(((((●)))))

Index

$(((((\bullet)))))$

About the Author

Wayne Perry's interest in the human voice, and ultimately spirituality and healing, was awakened at a very young age. He sang as a soloist in school choirs, studied voice with singing coaches, and performed with bands in clubs and concerts, eventually leading him to his inner voice at the age of 19. By age 22 he was initiated into the path of Sound Current Yoga, a spiritual practice that was to become his lifelong dedication. Wayne is inspired and committed to the soul of the voice and the voice of the soul.

Born and raised in Chicago, Wayne eventually directed his professional singing career to the West Coast and moved to Los Angeles in 1985. By 1991 he had produced and hosted several progressive radio shows. Through some of the interviews he conducted, he was led to the groundbreaking field of sound therapy and vibrational healing.

After researching and studying various sound technologies, Wayne founded the Sound Therapy Center of Los Angeles in 1993, the first sound healing facility of its kind in Southern California, offering private services, toning workshops, discussion groups, and sound therapy products. As director of S.T.C.L.A., Wayne has been in private practice as a sound therapist and vibrational healer, where his specialty is developing the profound therapeutic capabilities of the human voice. Using this methodology, he has healed himself of several health issues (including chronic allergies and kidney stones), and has helped to facilitate the healing of many hundreds of grateful clients.

Wayne's unique sound healing work has been featured on numerous local and nationally broadcast TV shows and radio programs. Since 1992 he has been producing and hosting *Wayne Perry's Heart Touch*, a popular, leading-edge television show discussing holistic health, sound, and spiritual healing.

Wayne has been a keynote speaker at various alternative health conferences, as well as a popular presenter at numerous mind-body-spirit events. He has also garnered international acclaim by conducting healing sessions, classes, and workshops in England, Italy, Egypt, and Japan, as well as in most major U.S. cities. In 1997, Wayne led an international group through a series of sound healing experiences throughout sacred sites in Egypt, culminating in personal healings for 65 individuals that he facilitated in the King's Chamber of the Great Pyramid of Giza. He has since conducted similar sacred healing ceremonies in Avebury, Glastonbury, and Stonehenge in England, and in Rome, Italy.

Highly regarded as a vibrational healer, teacher, and consultant, in 1993 he published "The Correlative Healing Chart for Sound Therapy," which is popularly used by healers and sound practitioners worldwide. In subsequent years he has created an assortment of sound healing educational products including comprehensive instructional CDs and DVDs, and several captivating music therapy recordings featuring only Wayne's remarkable voice and overtoning.

Wayne regularly conducts his Overtoning and Secrets to Sound Healing Weekend Intensive Workshop in Los Angeles and other cities. He also teaches the Professional Sound Healers Training Program.

Wayne lives in Los Angeles with his wife, Nicole.

For More Information
Seminars and Workshops

For information on Wayne's powerful and experiential Overtoning/Sound Healing workshops, seminars, and retreats, or if you would like to sponsor/host a workshop in your area, contact Wayne or Nicole:

> (800) A Sound He (800) 276–8634
>
> In California: (323) 655–7781
>
> Website: *www.wayneperry.com*
>
> Wayne@wayneperry.com
>
> Nicole@wayneperry.com

MUSIKARMA
Educational Products and Vocal Overtoning Music by Wayne Perry

> The Cosmichoir: Sounds for Self-Healing
>> 50 minutes/CD $18.95

InChantment

    59 minutes/CD $18.95

Remember the Future

    57 minutes/CD $18.95

The Secrets to Healing with Sound & Toning—A comprehensive, spoken word, instructional set of 4 CDs, containing toning and sound healing principles and exercises

    5 hours and 20 minutes/four CD Box Set $59.95

Prices are subject to change without notice.

All recordings are also available on audiocassette.

We accept Visa and MasterCard.

To order by phone:

    Call:

    (800) A Sound He/(800) 276–8634

    In California: (323) 655–7781

To order by mail:

    Send the full price of your order (California residents add 8.25% sales tax) in U.S. funds, plus postage and handling to:

    MUSIKARMA

    P.O. Box 48322, Dept. OCG, Los Angeles, CA 90048

Postage & Handling:

    For the U.S., Canada, and Mexico: $5.95 for orders of $20.00 and under; $9.95 for orders over $20.00.

    International Orders: Airmail: add freight equal to price of each book to the total price of order, plus $10 for each non-book order.

Allow two to four weeks for delivery.

Postage and handling rates subject to change.

≈

Visit our Website at *www.wayneperry.com* for information on additional sound healing products and services, and Wayne's speaking calendar.